The Heart's Truth

Literature and Medicine
Martin Kohn and Carol Donley, Editors

The Heart's Truth

ℰ

Essays on the Art of Nursing

ℰ

Cortney Davis

ℰ

The Kent State

University Press

KENT, OHIO

ℰ

© 2009 by The Kent State University Press, Kent, Ohio 44242

ALL RIGHTS RESERVED

Library of Congress Catalog Card Number 2008037051

ISBN 978-1-60635-003-4

Manufactured in the United States of America

The names and identifications of all patients, caregivers, and others mentioned
in these essays have been changed to protect their privacy.

LIBRARY OF CONGRESS CATALOGING-IN-PUBLICATION DATA

Davis, Cortney, 1945–

The heart's truth : essays on the art of nursing / by Cortney Davis.

p.   cm. — (Literature and medicine ; 17)

ISBN 978-1-60635-003-4 (pbk. : alk. paper) ∞

1. Nursing. I. Title. II. Series: Literature and medicine (Kent, Ohio) ; 17.

[DNLM: 1. Nursing—Essays. 2. Nursing—Personal Narratives. 3. Nurse-Patient Relations—

Essays. 4. Nurse-Patient Relations—Personal Narratives. 5. Nurses—psychology—Essays.

6. Nurses—psychology—Personal Narratives. WY 9 D266h 2009]

RT63.D348 2009

610.73—dc22

2008037051

14   7 6

I was visited by an angel in the middle of the night.
She stood like a nurse at the foot of my bed and wouldn't go away.
—ANNE MICHAELS FROM "FUGITIVE PIECES"

The most important practical lesson that can be given to
nurses is to teach them what to observe—how to observe.
—FLORENCE NIGHTINGALE FROM "NOTES ON NURSING"

For my children and my grandchildren;
in memory of my parents;
and for my patients

Contents

❧

Preface

While my grade school friends read *Cherry Ames, Student Nurse,* pretending to save their patients while at the same time wooing the handsome physicians, I'd jump on my bike and fly down the road pretending I might escape the world. Later, when high school companions talked about sacrifice and duty while thumbing through nursing school catalogs, I declared myself an art major. Packing my guitar, my black stockings, and my journal of poems, I went off to college, believing I'd escaped for real. Nursing, I told my friends, was not for me. I'd been hospitalized once when I was twelve, and that was enough. Forget the body and all its frailties. I longed to be an artist, a poet, to go beyond the flesh and connect with others soul to soul.

Then, somehow, I ended up right smack in the middle of the world I never wanted to inhabit, first becoming a nurse's aide, then a surgical technician, next a registered nurse, and, at last, a nurse practitioner. Along the way, I slowly discovered that nursing offered everything I'd thought only the arts could provide. I learned that there is nothing more personal or more universal than the experience of suffering, and that there are no words more significant than those spoken by a patient who has placed his or her life in your keeping. I learned that nursing is an odd, mysterious, humbling, addicting, and often transcendent profession, and that the reality of the body is the surest pathway to the mysteries of the soul.

What of my adolescent longing for drama and connection? The stories patients reveal—with their complex emotional and physical histories and the multilayering of their lives—are as entrancing and as important as the greatest novel. And ask any nurse about the duet played out by caregiver and patient behind closed doors. Together, a nurse and a patient experience a moment that is timeless.

I've been lucky—or maybe I've paid particular attention—but my desire to lead an artist's life has merged with my career as a professional nurse. Nursing has become for me, actually and metaphorically, that maternal place where the creative and the clinical intersect, where soul and body merge. I've learned that clinical time—those fleeting, difficult to describe moments with patients that, once played out, are unalterable—can be captured in creative time, and that what has happened *for real* can be recast in the imagination, in the poem, in the short story.

In these essays, I've taken a look back, examining again events in my nursing career that seemed to shake me, commanding me to pay attention. Nursing is full of such moments. Sometimes they occur in the bright light of the ward in daytime; sometimes they happen at the bedside and are gone in a flash. I hope that by writing about what I've experienced, I might illuminate the way not only for those students who want, more than anything, to become nurses but also for those who, like me, stumbled into nursing by accident or by necessity, unaware that the act of nursing would take their breath away—that their lives, and the lives of their patients, would be forever transformed.

The Other Side of Illness

I heard a woman say, *your operation is over.* I had been a long time waking. As I swam back toward the sounds of the recovery room, I was aware of hands touching my arms and adjusting what seemed to be an endless number of new appendages—tubes and wires that snaked from my body like bare branches on a winter tree. Ah, I thought. This one must be a nurse, the owner of the voice that's now saying, *good-bye, good luck.* Then there was a lurch and a floating sensation as my gurney was wheeled away.

When all motion stopped, I vaguely realized I was in my room. A centipede with a hundred hands lifted me from the stretcher to the cold bed. More hands rolled me from side to side, then a woman who smelled like soap enfolded me in a warm blanket, and I disappeared.

I hadn't been a patient for many years. In fact, just days ago I had been the strong nurse on the other side of illness. When I found myself lying in the emergency room, subjected to all those odious procedures to which I once glibly sent my patients, I was reminded of how thin the line is between health and sickness. How easy it is to feel *good.* How quickly we can give that up and fall helplessly into disability's deep crevice.

For the next several days, I wondered if I would live or die, at the same time chiding myself for such dramatics. I struggled to make sense of my symptoms, reassuring myself that the weird nightmares were due to the central nervous system effects of the antiemetics, that the nasogastric tube was indescribably uncomfortable because it was irritating my nasopharynx, and that the unremitting nausea was a hangover from the anesthesia. Whenever I floated to consciousness, I took inventory of my body, as patients tell me they've done: *Yes, my heart is beating. Yes, I feel pain, so I must be alive.*

I could rationalize my symptoms, but that clinical mastery did nothing to calm my fears. All the while, nurses came and went from my bedside, administering medications, changing IV bags, soothing me, and holding my hand when there was nothing else they could do. For the first time, I realized the importance—the impact—of this kind of consistent, nonjudgmental caring.

While doctors visited once daily and gave their brief pronouncements, nurses were ever present, comforting me and standing vigil over the workings of my body—the rise and fall of oxygen, measured by the clip on my index finger; the fluctuation of blood pressure and the ooze of fluid from my incision; the rewrapping of bulky antiembolic pads that whooshed and squeezed my legs all day and night. Those reassuring rhythms contrasted with the growing necessity I felt to hold on to what was *normal*. If one could recall what it was like to be a whole person, I reasoned, one could set a course to recapture that feeling. I also wondered if I was in this situation because I needed to discover what it was *really* like to be a patient. Perhaps I had grown too complacent after twenty-seven years in nursing and had failed to be as alert as I should have been. I decided that someone had found me out and sent me here for repair.

So I paid attention to what I saw and thought about in the dark. Sometimes I'd wake and see a nurse, like a dream vision or a cool drink offered in the midst of a suffocating desert, standing over me to adjust the equipment that kept my body in equilibrium. Then I understood what my presence as a caregiver must have meant to the patients I've tended.

I also gained a new appreciation of how suffering alters time. The clock on the wall glowed in the dim light. Whenever I looked, only minutes had passed, as if fear grasped the slender hands and held them back, magnifying every bodily sensation and dragging out every pain as if it were taffy, sickly sweet and stretched to the breaking point. As hours inched by, I realized how mortal and common I was— just one patient on a floor filled to capacity. Nevertheless, I was *me*. I reminded myself that every patient has a unique tale and their own, individual suffering.

Little by little I recovered, and as I did the nurses' routines changed. They lingered to talk. They fussed over my flowers, snipping off withered blooms and tipping cupfuls of water into the vases. They made sure I had everything I needed: my comb, my magazine, the call bell pinned to my johnny coat. They entered my room less often, and whole nights went by without their disturbances.

A day before my discharge, they moved away from me completely, setting me free just as a mother lets go of her grown child. This progressive separation was, I realized, a dance as well-rehearsed as a complicated madrigal. In the beginning, the nurses' actions intertwined with mine, close and magical. As I needed less, they moved away in ever-widening circles until suddenly I found myself dancing on my own.

This time of illness allowed me to look at my nursing role from another vantage point. All along, I had known how we caregivers move in and out of a patient's grief or happiness, changing our expressions, lowering our voices, going from one room that is blessed to another that has gone cold as January. Like others, I've collected the stories—patients blasted with disease who should have died but didn't; healthy patients who died anyway, perhaps not of a broken body but of a shattered heart. Now, more than ever, I understood how someone might will themselves to die, or how, to a point, patients could will themselves to live.

I also learned how caregivers' and patients' experiences intertwine. For that terrible, suspended time of illness, patients sink into our care wholly and confidently. They let us carry them. They come to know us—not the secrets of our lives, but the intent of our hearts—as intimately as we come to know the details of their flesh. Today, healed and returned to the land of the healthy, when I stand at a patient's bedside, I see my actions through their eyes.

The sense that my illness served as a warning lingers. *Pay attention nurse!* it says. *What you do and who you are when you care for a patient is significant. Your presence etches a chapter into the story of each patient's life that can never be erased.*

Washing Mrs. Cardiff's Feet

On a sunny, late February day in 1970, I knelt for the first time ever to wash a patient's feet. She was a fifty-five-year-old woman in heart failure who would die less than a week later. I was in my first year of nursing school.

I washed Mrs. Cardiff's feet at Saint Joseph's Hospital, a community institution commandeered by Sister Mary Margaret, a tiny, middle-aged nun in voluminous black who moved silently through the wards, always appearing just in time to correct a near error in patient care or to catch a sloppily tightened draw sheet. At St. Joe's—what we students and many of the nurses called the hospital—most patients lingered in wards, four or five beds along one wall, an equal number against the other. Green fabric curtains on squeaky metal rings surrounded the beds, allowing only sounds and smells and the silent vibrations of sorrow to penetrate their borders. When all the curtains were opened, as they were at night and for meals, the two rows of patients faced each other like chess pieces. Upright and fragile in their johnny gowns or lying on their scratchy bleached sheets, every patient knew what was wrong with, and what was happening to, every other patient.

Walking through Sister Mary Margaret's halls, I tried to assume the demeanor befitting my new student nurse's uniform: a white-collared striped blue dress, cinched at the waist with a tuck that held bandage scissors and a small clamp, called a mosquito, that was handy for twisting off IV bottle caps and performing other mysterious, as yet unlearned, tricks of the nursing trade. We students went bareheaded until our second year when, after an elaborate ceremony, we each sported a pure white, high-winged cap with one pale blue velvet ribbon. The second ribbon, dark blue, would come only with graduation. I didn't yet know that along with graduation would come an assortment of grave responsibilities. I would come to understand this because in my first year of nursing school I was—first with reluctance, then in gratitude—called to wash Mrs. Cardiff's feet.

She'd been placed not in the women's ward but in one of the few semiprivate rooms. The bed by the door was vacant, its occupant off somewhere for a test or an operation, and so that first day it was just Mrs. Cardiff and me in the small, antiseptic-smelling room. Sunlight, the cold glow of midwinter, filtered in through the one window overlooking the parking lot. Transformed by its passage through glass and over the forced hot air hissing out of the radiator, the sunlight warmed the bed on which Mrs. Cardiff reclined, her hair dyed blond and done up in the stiff, poufy style of the day. She wore her own nightgowns, refusing the thin, limp hospital gowns, and, with a less-than-steady hand, she applied mascara and a touch of coral lipstick each morning. She was unwilling to give up on the *self* she held in her mind's eye because if she did, she told me, she might slide into the black hole of illness. She wasn't ready to let go of her husband, her son, her grandchildren.

Reading her chart, I had some idea of the actual desperation of her condition. Twenty years before she'd been diagnosed with breast cancer and survived. A decade later, unrelated to the cancer, her heart began, insidiously, to rebel. Now it was twice normal size, its maintenance dependent on a long list of medications that I scrambled to look up before administering: medicines to steady the ventricle that was prone to go into fibrillation, a disorganized quivering, and tablets that drew unwanted fluid from her tissues and dumped it into her veins, rushing it through to her kidneys. Without these she could, in an eye blink, go into heart failure. It seemed, from the physician's note, that Mrs. Cardiff might expire at any moment. Standing before her that morning, her chart clenched in my hand, the light playing over her golden hair and vibrating the dust motes between us, I wondered if she sensed her fate.

In my mind's eye, I pictured what I might do to save her if, right before me, her heart stopped. I would pull her from the bed to the floor, place the heel of my hand, fingers locked, over her sternum and, calling *Help! I need help!* pump her heart back to life even before the nurses arrived. Maybe she would stop breathing and I would be the one, alone in the room with her, to grab the Ambu bag, place it tightly over her mouth and nose and squeeze the bag, filling her lungs, turning her dusky skin rosy again. Part of me wanted Mrs. Cardiff to get better and go home. Another part of me wanted *something* to happen so I could save her.

I introduced myself as the student nurse who would care for her over the next few weeks. She smiled, as if resigned to the flow of nurses and aides and interns and students who came and went from her bedside. Eager to assess her skin for cyanosis, her jugular veins for distention, her extremities for edema, I said I'd get things ready for her bath. But she stopped me to say that in fact she had already sponged herself earlier that morning. She pointed to the green plastic bath basin on her bedside stand. The now-cool water's surface sparkled with cast-off skin cells, filmy evidence of the body's never-ending quest to renew itself.

Never mind then, I said, and proceeded to clean up. I emptied the bath basin, wrung out her washcloth, gathered her barely damp towels, and returned her toothbrush, toothpaste, glasses case, deodorant, perfume atomizer, and satiny makeup kit to the bedside stand's single metal drawer. She asked if I would fetch her a clean nightie from the closet—her husband brought them in daily—and help her slip off the old gown and slide into the new. In the process, I caught a glimpse of her chest with its absent right breast and the pale, ladder-track scar that marked its place. I saw the wide, ruddy scar that split her sternum into *this side* and *that side,* the aftermath of the several surgeries she'd required after her several heart attacks. She'd been ill almost as long as I'd been alive.

I asked if she was ready to get out of bed and sit up for a while.

Yes, she nodded. She'd like that very much.

A fresh white sheet, snapped and billowed open, made the dust motes fly. I smoothed the sheet over the chair and tucked it in. Slippers for her feet. Head of the bed cranked up with the worn steel handle that, when the cranking was done, folded back underneath the foot of the bed. I helped her to a sitting position, guided her legs and then her oxygen tubing over the edge of the mattress as the sheets crumpled beneath her and slipped down from the head of the bed to expose the bare gray mattress. The sunlight now in her eyes, the room warm, Mrs. Cardiff lingered somewhere between conversational and pensive, moving back and forth between these two states according to the effort needed to stand, to swing around, to sit again in the chair. She arranged her nightgown. I bent to reposition her slippers. Next I checked her pulse. Although part of me anticipated crisis, at the same time I found it almost impossible to believe that she could die. She looked so alive. So *embodied.*

"Wait, dear," she said, and extended her hand. I looked up. My uniform was stiff and crisply ironed. My Clinic brand nurses' shoes were polished, classic.

"Would you wash and lotion my feet?" Mrs. Cardiff asked. "That's the only part I can't reach."

I paused. Wash her feet? But what of her pulse rate, her respirations, her blood pressure monitoring, all the *real* nursing tasks I might do? What about CPR, *extreme means?* Mrs. Cardiff looked at me, eyes bright, hand still outstretched as if to stop me before I vanished like all the others.

"Of course," I said. "I'd be happy to."

I tallied the required essentials and then, from the linen cart in the hallway, plucked clean towels, one to kneel on, two to dry each foot separately. From the top of the cart, I selected a Chux, the blue plastic-backed pad that I'd place under the washbasin on the floor. Balancing my armload, I returned to the room where Mrs. Cardiff, perhaps thinking herself for a moment unobserved, rested with her head fallen back against the high rim of the chair, her face turned to the sun. I could see the movement of her heart, a twisting so violent it shook her left breast and the nightgown that covered it. Her breath came in soft, pursed-lip exhalations, as if she'd run a long distance and now paused, exhausted, in the chair. The bright light accentuated the marks of pain across her skin, the creases that come with grimacing and, after a time, do not go away. When she heard me, she turned. Her face moved again into shadow, and the marks disappeared.

I put my supplies down on the over-bed tray and went to fill the basin with almost-hot water, knowing how quickly it would cool once exposed to cloth and skin. Finally, I knelt before Mrs. Cardiff, slipped off her paper scuffs, settled the steaming basin, and gently lifted her right foot into the water. Maybe later I would save her by administering CPR with skill and style. For now, I thought, at least I'd do a good job of washing her feet.

"How's the temperature?" I asked, knowing already—my nurse's instinct honed far in advance of my technical skills—that it was just right.

Her foot paled and changed shape as it submerged, that visual trick of the body's continuity broken by the water's surface. "It's perfect," she said. My heart offered up an extra beat, a strong *poom poom* that interrupted the regular sinus rhythm of my pulse. That was my heart opening. Or at least that's what I think now, looking back.

Silently, I took the washcloth and tri-folded it around my right hand, wet and soaped it. Then, cradling her foot in my other hand, I washed. Her foot was narrow and veined, perhaps a size 6, with a high arch and a bunion that forced her great toe to tilt in a bit, causing a tiny callous I could feel between the great toe and the second toe. I washed firmly and slowly, rinsed, let the foot go back into the basin, becoming pale and otherworldly again. I wanted to dry her foot, change the water, proceed on to the left, but Mrs. Cardiff would have none of it. "Oh," she said, "Let's soak them together!" She let me de-slipper her left foot and bring it to rest in the basin next to her wrinkly and already waterlogged right foot. I watched her feet settle gray and luminous under the water's meniscus. She wiggled her toes, sloshing the water. Or perhaps her toes, little doughy appendages, were simply vibrating with each heavy contraction of her heart.

Having her feet washed gave Mrs. Cardiff immeasurable pleasure. The other things I did for her—bringing in her medications in their little fluted cups; measuring her blood pressure; helping her walk a few steps to the commode (an effort that left her gasping), then wiping her, measuring and emptying her urine into the toilet; adjusting and readjusting her nasal oxygen, the green plastic tubes that irritated her nose and piqued her sense of independence—none of these ministrations helped her, she said, as much as washing her feet. And so for the next four days, I returned to Mrs. Cardiff's room and, our ritual established, silently knelt before her. There, I learned something about caregiving that none of my professors could teach me. Mrs. Cardiff introduced me to the laying on of hands—those ministries that may include the heroic but more often include the humbling, the mundane, and even the seemingly unnecessary.

When I returned to St. Joe's the following week, I was assigned a new patient. Mrs. Cardiff had died on Saturday, the day after I last tended her. The nurses and doctors had pounded her chest, forced oxygen into her lungs, shocked her heart, and used every medication they had, but nothing worked. Perhaps we should have, but Mrs. Cardiff and I never spoke about the possibility of her death. We said nothing about the past or the future. Leaning back in her chair, sometimes dozing, Mrs. Cardiff existed only in the present: her husband's visits, new pictures of her grandchildren, the intimate daily ritual of washing her feet.

For me, this ritual had been at first simply a menial task, a job I performed while waiting to do something more significant. As a graduate nurse in intensive care, I would soon enough have my share of heroics. I would give mouth-to-mouth resuscitation to a dying man. I would stop a hemorrhaging woman's blood with my hands, splattering her face and my own. I would strip away burned flesh from a young boy's legs. But as my week with Mrs. Cardiff went on, bathing her feet became an important act in itself. I came to understand that such simple acts of caring may not restore the pulse or bring back the breath, but they do, in their own gentle way, save lives. Although we are, all of us, more than our bodies, it is *in* our bodies that we exist on this earth. It is at the borders of our bodies, skin to skin, that we connect, love, praise, and serve.

The Evening Back Rub

When I was a student nurse, I perfected the art of giving a great back rub, a skill I'd first learned as a nurse's aide. In my second year of nurses' training, when we students worked evening shift, I'd gather my equipment and push my cart from room to room, checking IVs, changing rumpled sheets, offering fruit juice with crushed ice, and giving every patient a back rub. For most patients, this quiet ritual brought relief from boredom and loneliness. For me, it became a private interlude during which I could listen to patients tell their stories or admit their fears. While my hands massaged their backs, patients could escape, at least temporarily, the hospital's stark walls and the day's long hours.

This is how it went. After taking a patient's blood pressure and checking the pumps and monitors that hummed monotonously in the background, I'd draw the curtain, crank up the bed so I wouldn't have too far to bend, and help the patient turn on her side. Next I'd fanfold the sheet to expose her back, the muscles tense, skin red and ridged from the pressure of the bedclothes. Sometimes, a patient's ribs stuck out like ladder rungs.

I'd snap open the bottle of lotion and pour a little pool of it into my palm, warming it in my hands until the scent of almonds drifted into the air. Alone with my patient in the half dark, I'd slather the lotion from shoulders to buttocks, gently swirling my hands in long strokes until the entire back was slick and soft. After a minute or so, the patient might begin talking, and I'd gradually increase my fingers' pressure until I was rhythmically kneading the skin, increasing blood flow and urging the patient's body to let go, to trust me, to relax. I'd learned that a good back rub lasted ten minutes—ten minutes' attention to the flesh and soul.

Alas, nurses rarely give back rubs anymore. Time once devoted to patients is now spent requesting off-formulary medications or arguing with insurance companies about *why* Mrs. Smith should stay in the hospital for one more day. Now, instead of offering ten minutes of human interaction during which a nurse's hands might become a conduit of healing, we rush in and toss the patient a prepackaged, prewarmed washcloth. Those little bottles of almond lotion, once tucked into every patient's bedside stand, have just about disappeared.

A lot has changed since the days when I wore my blue students' uniform and patients recuperated in the hospital for weeks. Today I wear street clothes and a lab coat and only the sickest patients qualify for admission—and even they are sent packing after a few days, heads still spinning, bellies aching. No longer able to heal according to their own rhythms, patients are hurried along "critical pathways," insurance companies' predetermined timetables for recovery; we nurses, once our patients' advocates and masters of the evening back rub, mourn all that's changed and all that's lost from our noble profession. Some of my nurse-friends have left their jobs to find happier occupations. I read that, these days, fewer young women and men opt to pursue bedside careers.

As for me, I'll hold on to the memory of the evening back rub, that once-upon-a-time when a suffering patient could be comforted and I had time to linger and listen. Now when I greet a patient—before I verify her insurance plan and check to see which treatments she may or may not receive, and before I determine how much time I'm permitted to spend with her—I place my hand on her arm for a while and we talk. Just for that moment, the years roll back and there is nothing and no one between us, as it should be.

Being at the Bedside of the Dying

If you work in our field long enough, no matter where you're employed or where your ambition takes you, sooner or later you will be called on to sit with the sick, the grieving, and the dying. Some of us, those who do our nursing in places like the intensive care unit or the cancer ward, perhaps sit with the dying and the grieving more often. Never mind. Sooner or later, this task comes to us all.

The first time I saw a dead person I was a nurse's aide, my first evening on the job. The charge nurse had asked me to make vital signs rounds, going from room to room and taking the patients' temperatures, pulses, and blood pressures. I set off with my clipboard and a stethoscope, feeling a bit awkward in my new blue uniform and white shoes, scissors tucked into my pocket. At first, everything went fine. I introduced myself and chatted with patients, some in double rooms, some in eight-bed wards. I'd take a patient's glass thermometer from the bedside plastic holder, wipe off the alcohol (I can still smell the sharp, white smell of it), shake down the glittery column of mercury, and place the glass rod under the patient's tongue. While the thermometer "cooked," I held the patient's wrist and counted the heartbeats for one minute. Like most of the other aides, I fudged on the respirations, writing down "20" for each patient. It wasn't until later, when I became a nurse, like the nurses around me that first night—the women in white, the ones who soothed patients with a word or a gesture, the ones who knew how to insert intravenous lines and how to shock patients back to life—that I realized twelve breaths a minute was the norm.

Odd, then, that it was Mr. Tonelli's obvious lack of breathing that first caught my attention when I pulled back his curtain and called, "Good evening! Here to take your blood pressure!" My patient didn't answer. Flat on his back, eyes open and fixed on the overhead light, the old man's mouth was a round "O" underneath the overhang of his boney nose. Something was missing, as if whatever made him Mr. Tonelli had gotten up and left, abandoning the unbreathing husk of him, leaving it behind for me to find. His skin was gray, shriveled, and dry to my one-finger touch. In an instant, I recognized *dead.* Dead as my gerbil had been when I was six, dead as all those goldfish floating sideways at the top of the tanks of my childhood, dead as the puppy I'd seen hit by a car when I was ten. One minute, a body could be full and soft and illuminated by something that was, without a doubt, life. The next minute that same body could be sunken, inexplicably smaller, and dim, as if there indeed had been a radiant soul that was suddenly called away.

I stood for a moment staring at Mr. Tonelli. I stroked the freckled back of his hand. I felt his hard yellow nails. I touched his bare arm with the back of my hand, as if checking a baby's bath water. I leaned over to gaze into his eyes, blue and sunken into their orbits. I remember saying a prayer, something like, "Please let his soul ascend unto heaven and rest in peace." I took a deep breath, as if for both of us, and sat down next to him on the bed. I'd never met Mr. Tonelli before, yet I felt honored to be the first one to see him like this. It seemed important, and an intimacy beyond words.

When I left his room to walk back and deliver the news to the charge nurse, I was changed. I'd seen death, *human* death. And while this man's dead body had something in common with the other bodies I'd seen, it was astoundingly different. I told the nurse, and she seemed to cave in a bit, as if someone in her keeping had slipped away unaccompanied, and this brought her pain. Looking back, I know how many deaths she must have seen, how many bodies she'd bathed and wrapped and walked to the morgue, how many families she'd called or cried with. She straightened her shoulders. "Was this your first?" she asked.

It wasn't until later that I experienced the *process* of dying, the passage of a patient from this world to the next. Being present during the dying is not like coming in after. *After* is like emerging from hiding when the storm has already passed and everything is silent. Dying, especially what hospice nurses call "the active phase," is not always easy to witness.

Actively dying, patients may be awake, talking and twisting, sweating, apparently fighting. Or they might be semiaware, gasping for air, opening their eyes and staring at you at the very moment their hearts freeze midbeat and the billowing in and out of their lungs stops. Or they might be totally comatose, dying privately, without giving us witnesses any hint of farewell. After Mr. Tonelli, after I'd become a registered nurse, after I'd sat with a few dying patients, my experience with death seemed never ending. It was as if death recognized that I'd somehow earned my stripes, my license, my diploma in *being there.* And so death took every opportunity to call me back into the room. Death threw everything at me: the kind of final hemorrhage we call "bleeding out"; burned, broken, or drowned children; postpartum mothers, their milk just coming in, who died from ruptured aneurysms; old women who smiled when they departed, mocking death, enabling me to smile too. Let death do what it will, I told myself. It's my job; it's my calling *to stay.*

And stay I did, always afraid, always with my heart pounding so mightily that it might have pumped the blood for both of us, me and my dying patient. Sometimes I felt as if I would faint or become ill; sometimes I felt the presence of God. Sometimes I felt the room electric with spirits, and sometimes I felt that the dying person was paying attention, living every moment, dragging death out because being *here* was so precious. Other times I felt dying patients rushing to leave, gladly turning their backs. A few times, death felt dangerous and overpowering. Every time, I studied what was happening like a novitiate. I didn't know then for what I was practicing.

My mother died in 1991 in a nursing home bed at 9:30 in the evening. My father slumped, overwhelmed, in a chair near her bedside. I sat on my mother's bed, as I'd sat on so many patients' beds, holding her hand. The heaviness of everyone's expectations—my own, my father's, the floor nurses', who thought that because I was there, they could be elsewhere—weighed on me. Because I was a nurse, everyone expected me to be brave, to stay, to somehow orchestrate this moment for all of us. Certainly that is what I expected of myself. But this time, everything was different. *This is my mother,* I wanted to cry. I wanted to run out to my car or sit in the waiting room. I wanted the luxury of saying, "I can't do this." At the same time, I wanted to be there. *I can do this,* I told myself. *I've done this so many times before.*

I did stay, feeling, more than ever, terrified, humbled, and unprepared.

Some years after my mother's death, I wrote about her dying. I was at last able to give voice to the division I'd felt at my mother's bedside, part of me her daughter, part of me a nurse. Perhaps it was this division that enabled me to do what I knew so well: to stroke my mother's hair, to recognize the final heartbeat, to say, over and over, that we were present, that we would walk with her all the way. In my writing, I tried to put into words what it's like for any of us to be there at that exact moment, the one we all think about, the one that can terrify, the one that can release. I wanted to say how difficult it is to be both caregiver and family member, both experienced at death and yet newly come to its bedside.

Something else happened in the process of writing about being present at my mother's death. I let go of much of the terror that being in the presence of the dying can awake in me. I began to see beyond the many individual deaths I've witnessed to the greater arc that we call the life cycle, that continuous coming and going, and I began to *feel* the rightness of it, the comfort of it. I began to see how all my patients, my parents, my loved ones, myself, are a part of this continuum, a cycle, glorious and spinning, that goes on forever. I came to trust what I had seen in so many dying patients' eyes, in their gestures, in the way their skin became luminous. Because I could believe that dying was not an end but a new beginning, I stopped believing in "death." I knew it was not the absolute finality.

I don't know if other nurses feel this way. I don't know if this is something that comes with age and maturity or with faith to all of us, or if it's only felt by those, like me, who've done their apprenticeships at the bedsides of the dying.

First Night in Charge

After completing my final year of nursing school, after taking my nursing boards and receiving the envelope that held my license, proof of my expertise, I became a real nurse in a real job: night shift in Intensive Care.

My nursing program had been a rigorous combination of clinical and academic work. By graduation, I'd run a floor, taken care of ventilator patients, started intravenous lines, passed meds, participated in codes, and, in general, was ready to hit the ground running. And so, after an eight-week heart-monitoring course, I found myself in charge of a seven-bed ICU, the only registered nurse on the night shift. I had a nurse's aide to help me, a woman in her fifties with thirty years of experience, and I had the support of the night supervisor who floated about from floor to floor, pushing the 3 A.M. snack cart, holder of the keys to the pharmacy and the morgue and the one to call in case of any emergency. But despite the aide and the supervisor, in that small unit of desperately ill patients, the buck stopped with me.

On my first night as charge nurse, I walked in to two fresh myocardial infarctions, an elderly post-op, and four ventilator patients, one of them a ten-year-old girl who had been hit by a car and was now dying. Was I scared? I was terrified.

But first, some background facts: everything was different then. The intensive care beds, separated by glass half-walls and long curtains, fanned out around a central nurse's station, a long desk where seven monitors beeped and pinged, echoing, a second behind, the rhythms of the seven monitors at the patients' bedsides, an odd, syncopated song that never stopped. There was an absence of computers and an even more curious absence of paperwork. An intake and output sheet hung by each patient's bedside; a nursing cardex held one page for each patient, and on that card was written a succinct nursing care plan and any important information about allergies, code status, and next of kin. Nurses' and doctors' notes were handwritten in the chart, available for all to read with a minimum of effort. And the change-of-shift report was given to the incoming nurses face-to-face, not taped or typed into a computer to be printed out and passed along like a secret note. In other words, we had a lot less aggravation and a lot more time to spend with our patients.

And spend time with patients we did. In intensive care there was no such thing as "rounds"—in our small unit, we were with our patients constantly. During the day, when most of the activity took place, there was a low patient-to-nurse ratio. Since we had no interns or residents, we nurses started and restarted IVs, placed or replaced nasogastic tubes, pushed curare to keep our ventilator patients sedated, and, because respiratory techs were not yet a common part of the team, we adjusted ventilator settings, ordered blood gasses, and then readjusted the vents to maintain doctor-ordered parameters.

Every patient was bathed once a day and "sponge bathed" in the evening, not with prepackaged and presoaped disposable cloths but with real soap and water. Each immobile patient was turned regularly, some every fifteen minutes. We gave back rubs three times a day, soaked and washed feet, got patients out of bed and hounded them to take deep breaths, to cough, to move, to mend.

Standing at the central nurses' station, I could see all my patients and, at the same time, watch their heart lines leap across the monitor screens in front of me. I could tell by a slight disturbance in the pattern when a patient was restless or having pain, and I knew that my duty was to go to that patient and help him. Sometimes *help* meant sitting by the bedside and talking; other times help meant recognizing an impending disaster, calling the attending, and positioning the code cart right outside the curtain, out of the patient's sight.

I'd done all these things and more as a student, always with an experienced nurse somewhere nearby. Even so, that first night in charge, as I walked in to that scene of illness and grief, I trembled as the evening charge nurse gave me report. I wasn't at all sure I would survive. I wasn't sure that I could help these patients survive and, more than that, was afraid I might harm them. I'd never felt more alone.

"Little Jennifer over there in cubicle three was hit by a car while riding her bike today," the evening nurse told me. "She has massive internal and neurological injuries, her blood pressure is dropping, they've got her paralyzed on a vent, and we still can't control her heart rate. The docs expect her to die within the hour, and her dad won't leave her side."

I looked over at cubicle three. A thin girl, sandy-haired, was barely visible in the bed. The respirator huffed beside her, and a spider web of tubes and catheters seemed to hold her captive. Hovering over her was a man with tousled dark hair, glasses, and a baseball jacket. He looked as if he had run from his house without money or comb, without anything in the world but his daughter, who now was in what we rightly call the agony of death. The father held his daughter's hand, and

I could hear him, his words muffled, as he pleaded with her to live. How could I, a new graduate—a well-trained one to be sure, but also one who didn't yet have the years of experience it takes to be a really good nurse—handle all this?

The evening nurses and aides and ward clerk left one by one, looking back over their shoulders at Jenny and her dad. As the automatic door whooshed closed, an eerie silence fell over the unit, interrupted only by the out-of-synch music of the respirators, each of them hissing its own tune, and the repeating voices of the seven monitors. The nurse's aide and I looked at each other. It seemed like only yesterday that I had been the aide, thinking that I could never be a nurse, never do what nurses were called to do.

"I'll take vital signs and make sure the IVs are okay," she said. She was probably just as frightened as I was, wondering if this new grad in her crisp white uniform was going to kill anyone that night.

I think maybe I did. I think I might have killed Jenny.

After all these years, I can't remember the exact sequence of events. In the middle of the night, when memory plays its tricks and dredges up the worst scenarios, the most awful implications, I think that I went to Jenny's bedside before I checked any other patients. I introduced myself to her father. I remember tears in my eyes as I watched them, father and daughter. I recall reading the medication cardex, the order for the intravenous medication to be given if Jenny's pulse exceeded a certain rate. I remember her wildly racing heart, suddenly well over two hundred beats per minute, and I remember drawing up the medication and administering it. Then, shortly after this administration, I remember Jenny dying.

It wasn't *then,* that night, that I wondered if I'd hastened Jenny's death. I didn't wonder this until years later, after I'd learned how human error and imperfect knowledge walk beside us nurses and doctors every minute of every shift. It wasn't until I'd had years of experience that I became familiar with how we caregivers can sometimes second-guess ourselves, especially when something goes wrong and we have to act instantly. That's when I thought of Jenny.

When I'm awake, feeling sure of myself and my skills, I recall a different memory. In fact, she didn't die within minutes of the medication but hours later. I remember that the night supervisor, a friendly, gray-haired woman, came to the unit to sit in the waiting room with Jenny's mother, who couldn't bear to be with her dying child. I remember this mother sobbing so violently that she was retching, a grief sound I'll never forget.

I remember that after Jenny died, her father insisted on helping me prepare his daughter's body for the morgue. I began to wash Jenny, and her father climbed into bed with her and took the washcloth from my hands. I started to remove her IVs and her father stopped me. "I want to do everything," he said, his eyes dry and dark, his voice firm. I stood back and watched as Jenny's father gently removed the tubes, the catheters. I helped as he wrapped her body in the plastic morgue bag, and I handed him the tags to tie on her toe and on the outside of the black shroud.

Did I kill Jenny? No, I tell myself. I know she was going to die, no matter what anyone did or didn't do. Instead, I tell myself that I learned a lot that night. One thing I learned was that sorrow comes when we least expect it, right in the middle of happiness. I learned most of all, perhaps, about grieving, about letting the survivors crawl into bed with their loved ones and *take part,* if that's what they need to do, or to let them, like Jenny's mother, get as far away as they want and *not* take part. I learned that we nurses, we caregivers, can be well trained and efficient and yet there will always be times when we doubt our actions. Did I, who thought she'd done it all by graduation, give that medication too quickly, bringing Jenny's heart to a crashing halt? Did I give it too slowly, and so not bring her heart rate down in time?

The rest of that first night in charge is now mostly a blur. I know that the other patients lived through the night, and so did the nurse's aide and I. The post-op patient voided, coughed, and sat in a chair. The other ventilator patients were suctioned, turned, medicated, bathed, rubbed, and talked to. The fresh MIs had no arrhythmias and received their medications on time. No IVs infiltrated or went dry. As dawn came to the unit, the sun arriving as a pale yellow line beneath the closed window shades, I sat with one man and talked to him about his family and his business. I watched as his heart rhythm slowed, steadied, helped by fifteen minutes of casual and reassuring conversation.

I can't tell you how many times in the years since that night I've looked up medications I'm about to give, their properties, their side effects, their benefits, and their dangers. I can't tell you how many times since then I've stopped myself before giving a medication or a treatment to check and make sure that what the doctor ordered was correct—doctors make mistakes too. I've learned that we caregivers are not infallible but only as human and sometimes as frightened as our patients. We're rarely as "in charge" as we may want to believe.

That long-ago night made me a better nurse; it taught me the need for abiding caution combined with confidence. Such caution has made me a safer nurse, especially today when everything has become more complex—how we do things, how we record things, how we interact with our patients and treat their diseases.

Still, I think about the small and mostly insignificant mistakes we can make, because we are human, every day that we care for patients—all of us, from the most famous and proficient doctor to the least experienced nurse's aide. No matter the reality of what actually happens, we caregivers always carry, along with our many responsibilities, the heavy and inevitable burden of doubt.

If we've ever done anything wrong, unknowingly, we can pray that our patients might forgive us. If we do make an error, we can admit it and ask our patients directly to forgive us. And when there is nothing to forgive, may we nurses keep away those dark imaginings and forgive ourselves.

Talking to No One

As I drove to work, a sudden snow squall sparkled and swirled in my headlight beams, illuminating the road ahead of me. *Beautiful,* I thought. Then I pulled into the dark mouth of the parking garage and the snow suddenly disappeared, the night closed around me. It was 10:45 P.M. In fifteen minutes I would begin my eight-hour night shift in Intensive Care.

Locking my car, walking into the hospital, riding up in the silent elevator, I brought the cold smell of *outside* with me. It clung to my coat, reminding me that there was indeed a world beyond the one that would now occupy my thoughts and my hands until dawn arrived to melt the dusting of snow that frosted the hospital walkway, the withered grass and the statue of Saint Joseph that stood just outside the main door. *Here* was work. *Home* was where my husband and children waited. Home was where, tomorrow, I would sleep while the children were in school; where I would dream about my patients. In dreams, their IVs would run dry, their hearts would stop, and they would cry out, startling me awake.

This was my sixth straight night in ICU. I was really, really tired and, never a night person, had been thrown off-kilter by the odd hours I had to keep in order to keep my job. Soon, I told myself, a position would open up on days. I'd been telling myself that for months. I knew that the night shift wasn't for me, but I knew something else as well. All these months on nights, I'd been honing my skills. I no longer trembled when the evening charge nurse gave me report. On nights, I'd been thrust over and over again into situations both critical and difficult. I'd had to use every bit of my training and every bit of my intuition.

The night shift aides now trusted me. The night supervisor came around less often, knowing that I would call her if needed. On my watch, patients received better care because less of my attention was spent learning how to be a good nurse. During all these nights, something had happened, slowly and consistently. Most of the time, I knew what I was doing. Mostly, I made good decisions.

I punched the silver disk that opened the doors to the ICU and the dim and silent hallway gave way to the bright, bustling ICU. Two nurses bent over a patient in cubicle six. A few aides scurried about finishing up their evening duties. The charge nurse sat at the desk running off monitor strips, her hair unraveled in curls around her face. I focused my gaze on cubicle five, for a moment holding my breath. Yes, there he was. Yes, the ventilator still worked its miracle, pumping oxygen into his lungs. Yes, his heart line still raged in great jagged spikes across the cardiac monitor suspended beside his bed. Joe had made it through another day. Now I would help him make it though another night.

Rita, the charge nurse, looked over and waved as I disappeared into the lounge to hang my coat and lock up my purse. I stopped for a moment in front of the mirror glued to the side of the locker and finger-combed my hair, bobby-pinned on my nurse's cap, its upswept white wings looking a little bit like a startled dove perched one inch back from my hairline. Then I went out to sit with Rita, pencil and paper in hand to get report. Mostly, I wanted to hear about Joe.

Why do some patients remain indelibly in our hearts and minds while others fade? Why do these few persist, living on in our thoughts and dreams? What was it about Joe that made him any different from any other patient I cared for during the long ICU nights? There had been others whose stories were more dramatic and whose illnesses more perplexing. There were some who'd been fun to care for, some I'd come to know well, and some who'd broken my heart. In contrast, Joe was almost a mystery. A fifty-nine-year-old construction worker, he was both a widower and childless. I didn't know if his parents were alive or dead in Italy, where he'd been born, and if he had any siblings, they never called or came to visit. He'd been brought by ambulance to the ER late one afternoon after a scaffold broke and he fell one story to the ground below. Unconscious, his brain swelling, he'd coded and then was resuscitated, put on a ventilator, and rushed to surgery. Afterward, when the neurosurgeons had done all they could, Joe had been brought to the ICU, where he remained. His brain either would or would not recover. In the meantime, he hovered between this life and the next, paralyzed by the curare we routinely pushed into his vein, medicine that kept him paralyzed, unable to fight the machines or move on his own.

What was it like, I wondered. Did Joe know that he was alive? Was his brain still functioning, his eyes still able to see even as his body was held captive, as if cased in cement, by the invisible chains of the medicine? What was it like to be *this* patient, waiting through the endless hours? Did he think? Did he dream? Did he hear me?

"Hey Joe," I said, going to his bedside after the evening staff had shuffled and chattered their way out of the ICU. With their exit, the commotion lessened and the *ping* of the monitors and the huffing of the machines became a rhythmic background melody. The lights were turned down a notch; the unit suddenly seemed smaller, more intimate. The patients, most of them unaware if it was day or night, nevertheless settled a bit deeper into their sheets and their hazy slumbers.

Joe was positioned on his back, arms at his sides, legs slightly bent, a foot-board pressed against the soles of his feet. He had a special mattress, one meant to relieve the pressure of constant bed rest, and he had two IVs, a nasogastric tube, and a central line. A catheter inserted into his penis drained his bladder; under his bed hung the Foley bag, a little purse that slowly filled, every shift, with bright yellow urine. Because he'd been on the ventilator now for more than two weeks, because the endotracheal tube had begun to erode the tissue in his nose and throat, the surgeons cut an opening into his trachea. Now the breathing tube protruded from his neck, cushioned by gauze pads and tied in place. Brown-haired, once muscular, Joe had, almost overnight, turned gray, and his body had softened, shrunken, devastated by the effects of prolonged bed rest no matter how often we passively moved his heavy legs, his floppy arms. Someone on the evening shift had taped his eyelids shut to keep him from staring, to keep his corneas from drying out and ulcerating. Joe couldn't even blink on his own.

While the aide checked the other patients' vital signs, I checked Joe's.

"Your blood pressure is great," I said. "And so begins another night. It's 11:30 P.M. on the ninth of December. It's snowing outside, not too heavy, just a quick storm. It was really beautiful driving in, like driving through a curtain of ice crystals—you know how it looks when the snow is rushing straight into your headlights?"

The ventilator bellows *whooshed* up and down, and Joe's chest rose and fell. "In ten days it'll be my daughter's birthday," I said. "Poor thing, she misses out every year. You know how when you're born close to Christmas some people decide to combine the gifts? Not fair, right? I did better by my son. He was born in August."

I checked Joe's IV lines and took a central pressure reading. "I'm checking your lines, Joe. Looks like Rita took good care of you this evening. I'll be back in a bit and we'll dance, okay?"

Joe and I "danced" every night that I was on. I'd put on the radio near his bed and, taking an arm or a leg, do passive range of motion exercises with him, sometimes humming and sometimes singing softly with the music, probably off-key, but I knew Joe wouldn't complain. Often I'd tell him the latest news. "And now, local and world politics," I'd announce. Then, while I emptied his Foley bag or changed an IV site or cleaned his trach or readjusted his position in bed, I'd mimic the newscasters and intone the events of the week. Joe had slept through local political scandals; he'd missed the rise and fall of the stock market; he didn't know that new apartments were going up downtown, buildings he might have worked on, and so I told him. Sometimes I waxed philosophical, asking

Joe questions about his state of being. I didn't ask him the great questions of life and death, although I thought maybe he was closer to the source of both and so might be more privy to the answers. *What do you hear, Joe?* I'd ask. *What do you think about all these hours? Do you sleep? Do you understand that you are alive, on a respirator? That you are healing and that we will take care of you until you do?* What I really wanted to ask was if he had glimpsed death, and if so, what was it like? Had he seen God? Had he seen heaven, even briefly, sparkling before him like an incredibly beautiful snowstorm?

The night crept along slowly and uneventfully for Joe, for me, for the aide, and for the other patients. It was good to have eight hours of peace in the unit; I had more time to talk to Joe and more time to spend with other patients. I told Joe I was really tired after all these night shifts. I told him I was looking forward to having three days off, days to go Christmas shopping for my kids and days to drink tea and read a book while they were in school and my husband was at work. I told Joe that he would be in good hands in my absence, although he might have to wait to hear the evening news or dance the rumba. Toward morning the aide walked by Joe's cubicle and laughed, pointing at me. "You're a hot ticket," she said. "Talking all these nights to no one."

When I returned after my days off, Joe wasn't in cubicle five. Instead an elderly woman curled in the sheets, a fresh post-op who would leave the unit by morning.

"What happened to Joe," I asked Rita.

"He got transferred to some nursing home in Westchester. The docs tried to certify him for more ICU time but couldn't, so they found a facility that took long-term vent patients. They moved him out yesterday." Rita knew I liked Joe; she knew I talked to him. She patted my hand and smiled. "He said to be sure and say good-bye."

I can't remember now how many weeks or months went by. I remember thinking about Joe, worried that he might be left to wither in the nursing home. I wondered if anyone danced with him or told him the news and the weather. I wondered if anyone had even told him what was going on, that he was being moved from the hospital to a nursing home. I wondered if Joe had died.

Then one night, right at midnight, a small man walked into the ICU.

He looked to be in his sixties, thin with a slight limp. I didn't recognize him.

"Can I help you," I asked, thinking he was a patient's husband or father. Who else would come at that hour?

"It's you," he said. "I recognize your voice."

I looked at him, smiling and all the time trying to place him. But didn't I know that face? A friend of a friend? An old teacher? A patient?

"Maybe I should lie down in bed and not move," he said. "Then we could dance."

"Joe?"

"Yes," he said. "It's me."

We hugged, a quick embarrassed embrace, our relationship altered now, forever changed. His face was open, happy, more creased than I remembered. It occurred to me that I'd never seen his face in motion, never seen him smile or heard his voice. The face I looked at night after night had been a motionless mask. Here before me, Joe was a different man. I wanted to call the aide who had mocked my rambling conversations. I wanted to say to her *see, all those nights I was talking to someone.*

"I came by to say thank you," he said. "You told me about the weather and what the doctors were thinking and doing. I heard everything. You held me to this life, you know."

I'm sure I had tears in my eyes. In reply, I said all the things we nurses are supposed to say: how wonderful he looked, how whatever I did was nothing, just a part of my job, part of the routine, what anyone would do, how happy I was to see him alive and well, how grateful I was that he had come to visit. What I didn't say is that I had loved him.

I'd gravitated to him as I had to few other patients. Maybe it was because he was so vulnerable and alone, in need of someone to talk to him. Maybe it was because I was young and still not that sure of myself, in spite of what seemed to be my growing confidence and expertise. Maybe, as I moved between the hospital world, where everything was a matter of life and death, and home, where I wanted everything and everyone to be safe, I felt as adrift as I imagined he felt. Maybe it was really me who needed him to listen.

Joe didn't stay long. It was late and he still wasn't, as he said, "quite a hundred percent." For a while we made small talk; then he told me about waking up, about the prolonged hours of physical therapy, about how his memory slowly returned. This time, I let him do all the talking.

"Now I've got to get going," he said. "You've got sick patients to tend, and I don't want to keep you."

As I watched him walk away from all those nights we'd shared, I knew I might never see Joe again. But what a gift he had given me. He'd taught me that when we nurses talk to an unconscious patient, no matter the cause of that patient's coma, we are never speaking to "no one." We're talking to someone who is cherished in this world, if only by the one nurse who chats, seemingly aimlessly, in order to make the hospital a less threatening place, to comfort someone who is suffering. We might never know if our voices are heard. It doesn't matter.

And I knew it didn't really matter if I ever saw Joe again; he and I would be forever in each other's keeping.

Nursing and the Word

Before we go any further, let me remind you that I *never* wanted to be a nurse. When other ten-year-old girls were somberly taking each other's pulses, playing at being nurses, I pretended that my Schwinn bike was a wild stallion. My imaginary cape flying, imaginary hoofbeats ringing out on the pavement, we galloped down Sylvandell Drive in Pittsburgh, always under the gray cloud of steel-mill smog that hung in the sky. When I was twelve, my father, a public relations writer, was transferred to New York City, and so we pulled up stakes, said good-bye to the smog, and moved to Stamford, Connecticut. I continued to ride my bike, but, alas, most of my new friends, like my old friends, thought about nothing but the day when they might become nurses. When we turned sixteen, many of my friends donned candy stripers' uniforms and gave of themselves at Saint Joseph's Hospital while I signed up for Saturday art classes at the local museum. After high school graduation, my candy striper friends debated the size, shape, and overall appeal of various nursing caps—their main criteria for choosing a nursing school—and I went off to Gettysburg College where I majored in art, joined the drama club, edited the literary magazine, and grew my hair down to the middle of my back. The thought of giving someone a bedpan or even a bed bath gave me the creeps. But life has a way of sending us where we never thought we'd go.

Move forward several years: I'm married with a baby daughter, and my husband and I are barely meeting the monthly rent. His cousin, a nurse's aide, suggests that I become a nurse's aide too: on-the-job training—at Saint Joseph's Hospital, of course—with flexible hours, uniforms provided, and, best of all, decent pay. Feeling somewhat up against the financial wall, I enrolled in the six-week course, got my blue uniform (eerily similar to a candy striper's garb), bought white stockings and white Clinic shoes, and went to work four evenings a week from 6:00 to 11:30. When I returned at midnight, all was quiet—the baby in her crib, my husband snoring in our bed.

My very first night on my very first shift, I was introduced to the world of nursing in ways I couldn't have imagined. I walked into the elderly man's room to take his vital signs and found him cold and dead in bed. Later that night, a patient's husband called me an "angel of mercy," and a woman told me how afraid she was, waiting for the results of her biopsy. While I changed her sheets and then walked with her in the hall, she wept. After, as I was tidying up, she caught my hand and told me how grateful she was for my care. The hospital, I quickly learned, was a different world, one where people suffered and died. In the hospital, there was an undercurrent of mystery, sensuality, spirituality—here, love and caring were primal, like the love between a mother and a child, with all that relationship's fears, longings, difficulties, and joys. When I gave a worried patient a bed bath, my hands soothing her skin, I felt the same difficult-to-define selflessness that I felt caring for my baby girl. Little by little, I began to *like* my job.

I began to understand that in the hospital, during all those intimate and critical moments between nurse and patient, the caregiver becomes the transparent *giver*, and the patient becomes the very real *receiver*. Sick or recovering, a patient, like an infant, is helpless to do anything but exist in the moment. As a nurse's aide, I found great joy and great peace in the smallest but most important interactions: offering a cold glass of water to a thirsty patient, holding a lonely old woman's hand or listening to a man talk of his life, almost over. When I returned home at the end of my shift, everything was more precious. Everything reminded me that this other world—the suffering hospital—existed always, twenty-four hours a day. If I woke at 3 A.M., I knew that while I nursed my baby, somewhere a nurse's aide might be feeding a patient, or a nurse might be giving a patient pain medication or saving a patient's life. When I walked through the hospital doors in my squishy shoes and my neat blue uniform, not knowing what I would find, my heart opened like a hand.

At home I let my long hair fly loose, wrote poems about my growing daughter and soon about my new pregnancy and then my infant son. I still played my guitar, now substituting lullabies for the folk songs of my college days. But in the hospital, I became someone else—a braver someone, a more humble someone. I liked this person. I began to love what she did, laying her hands on the sick, listening to their stories, and helping them in small, limited ways. I watched the nurses with awe and found them heroic, dedicated, capable. Never, I thought, never could I be one of them.

Move forward again. My son gets sick and has to be admitted overnight. My daughter needs eye surgery, twice. My husband takes our car and his clothes and moves west, detouring through Mexico to obtain a divorce. A position opens up in the operating room for a surgical tech, which means more on-the-job training and a better salary and so, of course, I sign on. A year later, masked and gowned, I'm a single mother slapping instruments into the surgeons' hands.

In the OR, I'm once again surrounded by human misery and human tran-scendence. A drunk man bleeds out at midnight as the surgeons and I frantically race to remove his lacerated spleen; patients, almost anesthetized, turn to look at me and stare into my eyes, the only part of me they can see, and I hold their gaze. When I walk out of the OR, my mask down, red marks on my cheeks from the mask's pressure, nervous family members watch me. They ask if I was in the room with the one they loved, their child, their wife, their mother. In the OR, colors and sights and sounds swirl around me. The colors of the opened body are lovely—the glassy pink intestine, the deep red of muscle, the pearly white of tendon and bone. At home, I write poems and they become more sensual, more aware of sounds and smells, the smallest nuances. Yet still, my two worlds—my world of home and poems and my world of work and hospital—revolve around one another, spinning in tandem like electrons, but they never collide.

Fast-forward once again. I've taken the advice of the surgeons who've said to me, "You're a good tech; you should become a registered nurse" and gone back to a local community college to do just that. My previous college credits lighten my load. I take some courses at night and then arrange to work evenings to free my days for my clinical experience. I become friends with one of the other students, and, in order to survive financially, she and her son move in to my four-room apartment. We both work part-time, different days, watching each other's children and then, exhausted, study until 3 A.M. We begin dating the two brothers who live on the second floor. By the time we graduate, I'm engaged to one of the brothers, and my friend and I can run a busy floor, care for ventilator patients, give injections, pass meds, and resuscitate a coding patient with our eyes closed. I step right into a night job in Intensive Care, and she becomes a psych nurse in a tough rehab unit. Our days of financial scraping almost behind us, my kids and I have our apartment to ourselves, and my blossoming paycheck fills the refrigerator and buys everyone new shoes.

My fiancé and I get married. We move to a house about an hour away, and I leave St. Joe's to take a new job, also in Intensive Care, in a bigger, busier hospital. Within a few years, I'm promoted to head nurse on the hospital's brand-new twenty-bed oncology unit.

Click forward again, through hundreds of days and hundreds of patients, all of them sick or dying of cancer. On the oncology ward I witness the most profound suffering and the most devoted caring imaginable. I was a good nurse before, but on this ward, I become a *real* nurse. Then one day one of my favorite patients dies unexpectedly. This death, more than any other that I'd witnessed—and there had been so many—shakes me to my soul.

She was exactly my age. Her children were the same ages as my children. She had dark hair and blue eyes and freckles like me. My nickname was Cory and hers was Toby, but over the long course of her admissions and discharges, the doctors kept mixing us up. Finally, we'd answer to either name. Watching her, it was as if I watched myself.

When she died, I was at her bedside. I wept as I prepared her body for the morgue, and for months, I couldn't put her out of my mind. All my years in care-giving, everything that I'd seen and done, all the patients who lived or died—all those memories and moments seemed to overwhelm me. I almost quit nursing, asking myself, *why bother?* How could anything that I did possibly make any difference? Again and again, I'd run head-on into the cold stone wall of suffering and death, but this time I was unable to shake off my grief and simply go on. I couldn't, hadn't, healed my patient. How could I heal myself?

I didn't know what to do with my grief, a loss I couldn't, it seemed, share with anyone. After all, patients died every day, and, as another nurse reminded me, Toby hadn't been, not really, a personal friend. Nevertheless, the loss I felt was palpable.

Faced once again with the task of making sense of the pain of separation, I dug out my old poetry notebook. In a short, simple poem I wrote what it was like for her to die—how her family hadn't gotten there in time, how alike our lives were, how thin the line was between her as a patient and me as her nurse, and how final her dying was. Writing about her death, I felt a sudden, inexplicable release. I had captured her last moment forever. She would be, in this poem, forever in my life. But I had also, in the writing, let her go. I had forgiven her for dying and forgiven myself for not being able to save her, for not being able to save so many of my patients. In the poem, I came to terms, in some way, with my own mortal-ity. I had been there for her last breath; someday, another nurse would be there for mine.

Writing this poem allowed me to discharge my feelings of personal sorrow and professional inadequacy in the face of illness. The poem became a way to let my patient go and, paradoxically, a way to hold on to her memory forever. Writing that poem also rekindled the mystery of writing for me. I was reminded that when you think you can't find the right words to say something, that's where poetry begins.

From that moment on, my work in nursing became, more and more, the subject of my poems. My poems became like nurses themselves, healing me and at the same time documenting my patients' lives in transformative ways. Poems reminded me that I *did* make a difference in my patients' lives.

This *making a difference* is a nurse's calling, our most important work. Making a difference is that "something" that happens between us and our patients, most often in secret. There are meds and treatments to give, catheters to be changed and IVs to restart, heart rates to monitor and pump settings to adjust. But all these are only excuses for us to have *personal* contact with our patients—to talk to them, to tend them, to listen to them, to *be* with them. Nurses and patients share a thousand unobserved moments; it is those important but invisible moments that patients, and their nurses, remember.

I remember once when I was the patient, rushed in for emergency surgery. What I recall most vividly from that time is the way the nurse held my hand while she asked me her hurried questions. She didn't let go, steadying me, until they rolled me away on the gurney to the OR. That human contact held me together. A friend of mine remembers how a nurse, in the middle of the night, came into his hospital room where he lay, sweating and restless with fever. Silently, the nurse gathered water and washcloths and stayed with him, cooling his forehead, his neck, his arms. They never spoke, but he told me that he'd never felt more cared for, more loved in his life. When he bumped into her several months later at a local store, he burst into tears.

His tears were like my poems. They gave witness, gave voice to the way those nurses supported us by doing nothing heroic or especially technical but simply by performing compassionate deeds that no one else witnessed, moments that weren't recorded in the chart and that didn't show up on the hospital bill. Like my friend's tears, poems about my nursing interactions with patients can make those hidden moments visible and real. Poems or stories about my work capture those times and hold them in place; at the same time, they allow me to burrow beneath the surface of the moment, transporting me—and, I hope, the reader— beyond the individual experience to universal truths about life, suffering, and death. Poetry is like nursing and nursing is like poetry—both can change the world; both can heal and touch the deepest part of us.

Being a nurse helps me to be a better writer. Because I'm alert to the body's messages in health and disease, I can allow my poems to be sensual, replete with sights and sounds and noises and smells, with cries of suffering or songs of joy. Because, as a nurse, I'm engaged in the very human activity of caring for others, I can pour that reality into my writing, grounding what I do in the actual world and, at the same time, allowing what I do to be creative and open to imagination. In poems, I can change the endings that I cannot change in the hospital. In the hospital, I can encourage patients to talk to me, creating, in a sense, their own poems, a space in which to center their lives.

And being a poet helps me to be a better nurse. Because I have learned how to read and write poems on two levels, slick surface and deep metaphor, I can hear the story behind a patient's words. Because poems, the good ones anyway, are mysterious and transcendent, I've learned to be alert to the many holy moments that occur in caregiving and to accept them without embarrassment or doubt.

Poems help me to be creative, open, and more able to do what I must as a nurse. Poems, if we give our hearts to them, might prepare us all for nursing's most important work: paying attention; accepting; healing when we can; and when we can't, letting go.

Beyond Scientific Explanation

Strange things happen in hospitals, in nursing homes, at the bedsides of the suffering. Odd events become as routine to nurses as the daily tasks of monitoring and medicating patients or staying with them as they die, some struggling, others slipping away peacefully. Nurses understand that something beyond our human comprehension occurs when the last breath is expelled, the one that completes the cycle begun when the patient, as a newborn, took in that first, hearty lungful.

This last exhalation lets go not only the energy accumulated in the chemical processes of living but also the essence of what, to me, is evidence of the soul. The body deflates like a balloon with a pinpoint leak. Only the patient's eyes (which often remain open) reflect the drama of this change. The gaze wanders, first fixing on something nearby, perhaps a loved one in the room. The life spark, that moist glimmer we are so accustomed to, dims, as if a cloud has passed over. Then the eyes, once the arbiter of earthly sight, look away to focus on some other vision, one we in attendance cannot share.

Sometimes patients can see their fate arriving, like the elderly woman on the oncology unit who wouldn't unclench her fists for fear of releasing "Dr. Death," a presence she had trapped and now, terrified, didn't dare let go. But her nails were long, cutting into her palms, and so we good nurses pried her fingers open one by one, reassuring her all the while. After the last nail was clipped, her hands open, she sighed, resigned. "What's the use?" she said. "Now he's in the room." Moments later, she died. Watching her depart, we were humbled and afraid.

So what of ghosts? Although we often see the soul leaving the body, it's mostly what happens after death that surprises us. Once, after a young girl died on the evening shift, the charge nurse received a phone call. The caller, identifying herself as the patient's mother, asked that her daughter's body be held on the ward for a few hours, giving her time "to come and say good-bye." When I arrived the next morning, I was shocked to see the girl's body still in her room. I asked why she had not been taken to the morgue, and the night nurse explained that they were still waiting for the mother's visit. My heart skipped a beat and then became a steady rhythm that swelled into my throat, my temples. I knew what the other nurses did not know—that the patient's mother had died years before. When I told them, we sat for a moment in silence. Who was the woman who called, asking for a last chance to see her daughter? Was it the mother, and did she come to visit? We decided that she had and so prepared the girl's body for the morgue, carefully, lovingly. The nurses agreed that even if they had known that the mother was no longer alive, none of them would have ignored that phone call.

There are other stories of course: the way the elevator seems full of a swirling, dizzying "presence" for hours after we transport a body down to the basement morgue where the cold drawer waits, or the way some rooms seem forever haunted. A friend who works in another hospital says that every patient placed in a certain room always survives, even when, judging by the severity of their condition, they shouldn't. She's sure it's the intercession of a patient who died there years ago, a young man injured in a car crash who'd wanted desperately to live. His often-repeated vow, that he'd come back to help other patients, seems not to have been a deluded rambling at all.

My favorite story concerns Otto, a cranky, heavyset, chain-smoking guy who was our patient for weeks. Dying not of his cancer but of a superimposed infection, Otto rang his call bell persistently, stretching our collective patience to the limit. All day, Otto rang every fifteen minutes, the longest he could go without a nurse's voice or touch, something to remind him he was still a part of this world. When we went in to minister to him—to straighten his sheet or loosen his blanket or move his water glass—we would tease that we could set the clock by his calls. Some days, Otto's incessant demands drove us crazy. Some days, Otto's never-ending gratitude reminded us why we became nurses in the first place.

For two hours after Otto died, the ward seemed unusually quiet. Housekeeping came and cleaned his room, cranking the bed up high and stripping the linen, washing off the frame and the mattress, and then remaking it with clean sheets. They closed the door, and we all went about our business. Then the ringing began.

First we thought it must be a prank, someone pushing the call bell in Otto's old room as a hoax. We took turns going into the empty room to shut off the call bell, saying out loud, "Okay, Otto. Here we are." When the chiming persisted, we decided it must be a short in the wiring or a loose plug and called maintenance. A man in overalls replaced the call bell, even though he could find nothing wrong.

During the half hour of silence that followed, we breathed a sigh of relief and tried to convince ourselves that there was a scientific explanation, after all, for such an aberrant occurrence. But just at the change of shift, when nurses were counting medications and signing off patients to the oncoming staff, Otto's bell rang again. The bustle of activity stopped. We looked at one another, some of us frowning, most of us smiling. How silly to think, in such a miraculous place, that the answer was as simple as a frayed wire or a loose connection.

Five of us gathered in Otto's room. A few leaned against the wall. Some of us sat, as we used to, on the edge of his bed. We couldn't see Otto, but we knew he was there. One nurse promised she'd say hello whenever she passed the room. Someone else explained that we were getting busier now and needed time to spend with other patients. One nurse reassured him that it was okay to leave, that we were his family and we wouldn't forget him. That afternoon, the ringing stopped. By nightfall, another patient was in Otto's bed.

I don't work on the cancer ward anymore. After a few years there, I returned to school to become a nurse practitioner, first working in private practice, then in women's health, also places where strange and wonderful things happened all the time. Like most nurses, I'll always walk with ghosts. Like old friends, they come out to greet me—a reality I can't explain but find endlessly comforting.

Weekly Rounds

Another blustery January day, another Tuesday. Walking into the nursing home, I welcome the rush of warm air. At the same time, I recoil from the musty, antiseptic smell. I'm two years into my first job as a nurse practitioner in private practice with a group of physicians, and today's my day to do nursing home rounds. At the end of the afternoon I'll go back home, but right now I must go from floor to floor, seeking out our patients who linger here. After all my years in nursing, all my years going in and out of hospitals, I can't get used to this contrast: the world outside, bright and clear with the bustle of winter birds in the courtyard, and the sudden heaviness inside. Out *there* is sky and low clouds bringing snow. In *here* are the subtle odor of urine and the muted voices of the elderly patients, a steady low drone occasionally punctuated by a laugh or a cry.

Emma is first on my list today, a belligerent eighty-year-old woman who amazes me with verbal barrages that pack more zing than those of a longshore-man. I find her in bed, a rhinestone brooch pinned haphazardly to the bosom of her red nylon bathrobe. As I open the buttons to listen to her heart, I imagine the blood circling endlessly through the valves. "Watch it!" she shrieks when I palpate her abdomen, the skin loose and scarred with striae from six pregnan-cies. "The baby," she sobs, "you're going to hurt the baby!"

For a moment I ponder this bizarre scene: a tall, long-haired nurse leaning over a frightened old woman in bed. Perhaps she recalls the first cold probing of a doctor's hand sixty years ago. Or does she remember another scene, an in-sistent man's advances—or an angry husband's? I sit at her bedside. Sometimes I think my exams are pointless, done to fulfill the state requirements that regulate our nursing homes—rules that mean staff time must be spent filling out forms and checking boxes while patients are bound in chairs or lined up in hallways like old birds balanced on telephone wires, waiting. Yet I must be satisfied that Emma is not in heart failure, that the ulceration on her hip is healing, that her lungs do not rattle with the first suggestion of pneumonia.

"Emma." I say her name, and she gazes my way. Then, a burst of profanity.

"Emma!" This time, she sees me. "Hi," I say, and she grins. A connection! A current leaping across a rusty synapse! She pats my hand, a rough slap, like punching down dough or smacking dust from a horse's rump.

"I can't believe it," she says, shaking her head. "I don't even know where my house went."

We chat for a few seconds, just a flash in time. Then she is gone again, cursing someone who isn't there, someone who had the nerve to die before her. I leave the room and her voice chases after me. "And you'd better not forget!"

The day wears on. I look out the window, but the trees sway in silence, offering no consolation. I find Ruth in a wheelchair—Ruth who usually looks like a poker in bed, her head held at an angle inches above the pillow. Sitting upright, her crisp hazel eyes stare into mine.

"I feel just awful," she says. "Nothing I can put my finger on." Then she sighs. "This really isn't me, you know?"

Old Jim, a diabetic with one leg gone, pumps his wheelchair down the hall, an unlit cigar clenched in the corner of his mouth. He asks me to call his wife— she's two hours late. A nurse whisks by and pats his arm. "Today's Tuesday Jim. You know Helen only visits on Mondays and Fridays."

Jim removes his cigar. "It's not Friday?" He looks me up and down and sees Helen, thirty years ago. "You'll do," he says and asks for a light.

By late afternoon, all the names on my list are crossed off. I'm exhausted, feeling the creep of mortality. I wonder how long I would survive, tied in a chair, tapping my tray as the aides rushed by, impatient with me because I rebelled against the schedule: tub bath twice a week, music recreation at ten, "reality orientation" at eleven, where some young thing would tell me that today is Tuesday, cold and windy. That it's a new year in a new century. She would ask me, *what did you do for a living?*

At the elevator, I wait next to a woman dozing in her wheelchair, her head drooped forward on her chest. The elevator arrives, the door lurching open with a clunk, and she awakes, grips my skirt frantically as I step away, about to disappear.

"Let me die," she says. Then, level and direct, "Kill me."

I push the first floor button. As the door whooshes shut she raises her head and looks straight at me, memorizing my face, counting me among the many who have let her down. The door closes and I stare at the spot where I saw her last, the image of her eyes burned onto the metallic elevator door, the image of her eyes following me out to my car, driving with me through the dusk all the way home.

Inside my house the terrors overcome me. For the hundredth time, I vow to give up nursing—burned-out, fed up, sick and tired of sick patients. I could redo my resume, take up the cello, write full-time. Planning my escape, I let routine overtake me. I water my plants, snip brown leaves from the lush green with a surgical precision. Outside, it begins to snow.

But once Emma looked at me. "Oh!" she said. "Hi!" No cursing, no fist shaking in my face. Once Ruth told me about her children, laughed with me as she remembered their visits, their presents. Once old Jim told me how, as a younger man, he'd climbed a mountain in Africa. I water the last plant. The snow transforms the lawn from dark brown to white, and stars begin to blink into sight. I open the door and breathe. The cold air centers me. The appearance of the stars in their intricate patterns is a gift, so is the light touch of snow as it melts on my skin. And so is Emma's occasional *hi,* a brief recognition that the present exists and that my work matters. I step back inside and lock the door. Soon the moon will begin its slow climb and the stars will continue their dance across the sky, and I'll prepare for another day.

Twenty-four Hours in the Life of
a Nurse Practitioner

OCTOBER 7

2:00 A.M. Something wakes me—a dream? The house is quiet, and the yellow light from my husband's clock radio glows into the bedroom. I turn on my right side, wiggle my toes, and wait to drift away again. I tell myself I have to get some sleep.

6:05 A.M. The alarm goes off and a cold chill creeps through the covers. My husband yawns and gets up. I get up too, shivering. Today is one of my twelve-hour shifts in the women's health center, the hospital-based clinic where I've worked with the poor and underserved ever since leaving private practice. Twelve hours means three clinic sessions without a break. Already, I'm tired.

6:10 A.M. Standing in the shower, it takes me a minute to get oriented. I shampooed yesterday. I shaved my legs yesterday too. Funny how a woman will say, as she slides down into the stirrups for her Pap test, *I hope you don't mind that I didn't shave.* I say I don't even notice.

The bathroom steams up quickly. Light filters through the blinds, and suddenly I feel awake. And happy. The day will begin, and the day will end, a cycle over which, I remind myself, I have little control.

I say a quick prayer in the shower. There's something about this warm space that seems primal and exposed, as if here my soul might be as naked as my body. At the same time, I wonder if God objects to a woman who prays naked, soaping and scrubbing while she asks Him to protect her family, her friends, her patients.

Dry off. Get dressed: Black Victoria's Secret bra and black panties. Black slacks and an olive green slinky top. A slick of mascara and a line of brown pencil under my lower lashes. Professional on the outside, but inside I feel a little sexy. More like a poet—what I am on my days off—than a nurse practitioner. So this is what middle age looks like, I think, staring into the mirror.

7:00 A.M. While I eat breakfast, I reread a favorite book of poems, *Sloan Kettering,* by Abba Kovner, who wrote as he was dying of throat cancer. The poems are spare and wonderful. Suffering and blessings, endings and beginnings.

7:25 A.M. Out the door. If I'm lucky, if traffic hasn't picked up, if the school bus is behind, not in front of me, I'll arrive at the hospital by 7:50 A.M. As I drive through our neighborhood, I feel, viscerally, the seasons shift. The *feel* of the air has changed, reined in after the fullness of summer. In the sky, streaks of blue struggle to emerge from clouds. On the radio, the news, distant and personal at the same time: shootings, accidents, the ever-present clash of country against country, ideology against ideology. I try to imagine myself as victim, as patient. I remind myself to be kind.

7:53 A.M. I run up three flights from the parking garage to the women's health clinic, thighs burning. Have to do more exercise. Have to take care of my body. But when I enter the hospital corridor, everything—the rest of my life—is put on hold.

I clock in and walk into the back conference room I share with eight residents, another nurse practitioner, nurses, and secretaries—a room in which I have no desk, no chair, nothing but a drawer. I put my pocketbook into it, pull on my lab coat.

This morning is our monthly staff meeting. Afterward, I'll post myself in the hallway where I'll stand all day in between seeing patients. I check the schedule. Sixty patients due between 9 A.M. and 4:30 P.M. And another fifteen patients in the evening.

8:10 A.M. Waiting for the others to arrive, I call M., the coordinator of the hospital's Breast and Cervical Cancer Screening Program, and we talk about the latest abnormal Paps and mammograms. She shows me five reports, each one evidence of a problem that will require surgery, chemotherapy, or radiation. M. and I chat, both of us aware that these reports will change five women's lives forever.

8:15 A.M. Finally, everyone arrives: our supervisor, our medical director, the hospital's chief of OB-GYN (the only man here), our nurses, our secretaries, and the other nurse practitioner. First we praise the clinic's good work: more patients seen; charts more complete. The director restates her commitment to care for the underserved. It all sounds good, but the reality is we don't have enough providers or translators. There's pressure from administration because the clinic never generates enough money, and without money, resources are strained. Outside, a throng of women and children wait in the hall, all of them poor, most of them undocumented, each woman depending on us.

9:00 A.M. From now until noon, I lose track of time. Minutes here are measured only in patients and their stories. Our eight exam rooms fill up. I stand in the hall with L., the other nurse practitioner. There is one resident here too, a first year just learning her way around. She won't be much help.

My first patient, Sandra, is here for her initial pregnancy visit. She tells me she lost her first pregnancy at four months. "Will it happen again?" she asks. Calculating by her last period, she should be twelve weeks along, and we should hear the fetal heart. But when I place the doptone on her belly, there is only silence. I spend minutes searching. "Perhaps you're less pregnant than we think," I say. Then I track down the portable ultrasound machine.

On the ultrasound, I see a small fetus in my patient's uterus. It seems, every once in a while, to move, but I don't see the rapid fluttering of a fetal heart. There *is* a pregnancy within my patient's uterus, one much earlier than twelve weeks. It takes me fifteen minutes to arrange for Sandra to have an ultrasound in Perinatology in order to document, for sure, if there is a living pregnancy, if everything is okay.

The next patient is at the end of her forty weeks of pregnancy. Strong fetal heart. Baby's head down in the pelvis, ready and waiting. Nice, I think, to have this normal, easy visit. Maybe this will change the day's luck.

Then another pregnant woman, this one in the country for almost a year, comfortable with our American ways but still shy about practicing her limited English. She's thirty-six weeks pregnant and, after two previous C-sections, wants a third. "Otra niña!" she tells me, frowning. Another girl. I explain that we women can only reproduce girls. The father donates the chromosome that determines the baby's sex. My patient beams. This third girl is not her fault.

10:40 A.M. I've lost count of how many patients I've seen. I glance at the clock as I run to the bathroom for the first time. I've had nothing to drink since breakfast, no water, no tea, nothing. A patient waits in every exam room. We are really behind, some of it my fault. I took too long with my first patient, the one who's now upstairs having her ultrasound. Washing my hands for what seems the millionth time, I wonder if her pregnancy is okay. I'd asked her to come back and let me know.

I quickly see more OB checks, Pap tests, infection checks—then a seventeen-year-old who is twenty-six weeks pregnant, abandoned by her boyfriend and recently dropped out of school. She's depressed, losing weight, out of money, and at odds with her parents. I call the social worker. Some patients know how to navigate the system and get help. Others, like this teen, are lost and vulnerable. But, by the time the social worker finishes her intervention, the patient is smiling. The high school will take her back. After delivery, she can bring her infant to the school's babysitting facility; she can get state assistance. Her life begins to look a little better.

11:45 A.M. Lunch: peanut butter and jelly on whole wheat. Milk. A little Kit Kat bar from the bowl on the secretary's desk. I eat junk food at work that I'd never eat at home: chocolate kisses, jelly beans, a large Pepsi, and, sometimes, the wonderful almond pastry that the coffee shop sells for $2.85. On a busy day, I eat because I'm stressed. On a slow day, I wander between patients, searching for comfort food.

The clinic is not an easy place to work, and the lunchtime atmosphere is often edgy and negative. The nurses complain about the secretaries and the secretaries complain about the nurses. Whoever is out of the room is fair game. We talk about the previous clinic director who resigned (probably couldn't stand the craziness, we say) and the chief resident who's never around. Then we get up and walk back into the hallway.

12:30 P.M. Our afternoon resident is stuck in a difficult surgical case. Her ten patients will be added to our schedule. Much grumbling from the nurses who must now handle three full-to-the-brim columns of patients, a name in every fifteen-minute slot. Grumbling from L. too. She and I are the only providers here to see all these patients.

The first chart of the afternoon belongs to a pregnant woman who thinks her water has broken, although, for now, she has no contractions. As I walk into her room, I hear a secretary's voice rise up from the front office. "No more add-ons!" she shouts. "We don't have any more room!"

I've learned that the only way to get through the day is to keep moving forward. If I focus on one patient at a time, I can be completely *there*. But if I let myself think about the number of patients waiting or the evening clinic or the fact that I won't pull into my driveway until 8:45 P.M., then I'll be overwhelmed with that anxious, it's-all-up-to-me feeling, forgetting what I understood this morning—that I have little control. I can only take care of myself and the patient I'm with. Right now, it's this woman and, yes, her water has broken and she's about to go into labor.

1:00 P.M. My patient from this morning, Sandra, returns grinning from Perinatology with a copy of her ultrasound. Her pregnancy is fine but six weeks earlier than her last menstrual period would suggest. I admire the ultrasound picture: a tiny fetus with a yolk sac next to it, like a chick in an egg.

Patients arrive in fast succession. One is a woman whose last baby was delivered by C-section. This time, she wants to try a vaginal delivery, but we don't know what kind of uterine scar she has. Even if her belly scar is horizontal, there's a chance the internal uterine scar could be vertical, increasing the risk of uterine rupture. I tell her we have to request her old records, and, after her exam, we walk over to Medical Records where we get passed from one clerk to another, then to another office in another building. There, they tell me to request the records myself. I make a mental note to do this later. Back in the clinic, one of the nurses, D., tells me I have the patience of a saint. I disagree. I feel like exploding.

Patients all around me. A postmenopausal woman complains she's not able to hold her urine. The chief resident is supposed to see her to discuss surgery, but the resident arrives late and then lingers too long in the conference room. The patient storms out, angry. Sometimes, patients find the clinic overwhelming or humiliating—the noisy, multilingual chatter; the loud TV; people joking outside the exam rooms; rotating providers; the reality that the clinic is for the poor, the underserved.

In the next room, there's a thirty-four-year-old woman who's found a small lump in her right breast. It feels like a cyst, not a cancer, but I've learned to be cautious. I send her for a breast ultrasound, telling her that any mass, even one that seems benign, has to be investigated. I think of my friend, J., who just finished radiation for a breast cancer that came out of nowhere—a few microcalcifications on a mammogram, no lump, no family history. A biopsy found ductal cancer, early, well-contained, and treatable.

2:15 P.M. A pregnant diabetic is next, someone who should be seen by a senior resident, but there's no senior resident here so I pick up her chart: blood sugars out of control, a bladder infection. Her belly measures larger than her thirty weeks, and she still hasn't gone for diet counseling. I examine her, make phone calls to the dietician and visiting nurse, increase the patient's insulin dose, write a script for an antibiotic, and, of course, the resident appears just as I'm finishing up. Behind schedule again.

2:45 P.M. When I pick up this chart, I groan out loud. The nurse has written "patient severely depressed" in her note. This means, I know, a long and complicated visit. There are patients in every exam room and even overflowing the waiting area. Babies cry, women gossip in different languages, secretaries shout, nurses stand in the doorway and bellow patients' names at the top of their lungs:

NA-O-MI PHIL-LIPS! AN-TON-I-A SAL-A-ZAR! Leaning against the wall, I review the chart: a twenty-nine-year-old woman from Nepal. Postpartum seven weeks and crying all the time. Not suicidal. Husband translating.

The husband holds their newborn son while my patient huddles on the exam table, glassy-eyed, the sheet tied around her like a shroud. She keeps saying something in a reed-thin voice, but her husband won't interpret for me. I ask a question, he answers me. I stand with my hand on his wife's shoulder, trying to break down the wall he is building by his refusal to be our go-between. Finally I almost shout at him, "She keeps saying the same thing over and over. If I don't know what she's saying, I can't help her!" He looks at his wife and shakes his head. "She says she needs someone to take care of her."

I spend half an hour with them, going nowhere. I exam her and, physically, she's fine. But she's always crying, not sleeping, and barely caring for their newborn. When her husband looks at her, she flinches. To me, she has all the hallmarks of an abused woman but no obvious bruises. What does she do all day? Is she ever allowed to ask or answer questions herself? I consult with the social worker who takes my patient to crisis intervention. On the way out, the patient's husband holds her arm, tight.

3:30 P.M. Just when I'm sure there can be no more surprises, I pick up the chart of a thirty-five-year-old woman who is forty-one weeks pregnant, one week overdue, and here for her *first* prenatal visit. Maybe she has no money and so thought if she couldn't pay, she couldn't be seen. Maybe she doesn't understand the benefits of prenatal care. Maybe she wondered if the baby was ever going to arrive and so finally came in to see us.

She's my one and only English-speaking patient of the day, so at least I can go more quickly through the first-visit requirements: history, physical, lab tests, Pap, cultures, ultrasound, and all the testing and teaching that, normally, are spread out over forty weeks. And I have to discuss this patient with the chief resident. If we let this woman's pregnancy go on any longer she'll be at risk for a host of problems, including fetal demise. I want to scold her, *what were you thinking?* but don't. She goes off to the lab, request slips in hand, and says she'll come back in two days for induction of labor. I wonder if she'll show up. Then I remind myself to be kind.

4:00 P.M. The weekly high-risk conference begins in our back room. I'm still seeing patients so can't attend, although I'm supposed to. The residents who have been invisible all day suddenly appear. The door closes, and the residents and the Perinatologist discuss all the high-risk obstetrical patients, most of them seen by L. or me. She and I grumble once again in the hallway. We both just want to sit down.

4:55 P.M. Our evening clinic begins in five minutes, but I have to grab a snack before I can see one more patient. In the coffee shop, I get a glass of milk and a chocolate chip cookie "to go," mentally yelling at myself. Half of me says it's my reward. The other half says no wonder you can't lose that five pounds. I'm halfway through my cookie when the secretary says another add-on patient has arrived. We're on a treadmill that someone keeps speeding up. Deep breath. Only three more hours to go. Then I'll go home and make dinner, moving from one job into another.

5:05 P.M. As the evening schedule begins, the clinic atmosphere changes. Only L. and I are here with D., the nurse, and one secretary. The waiting room is full but not frantic. Someone turns down the volume on the TV. The phone hardly rings.

Although I'm exhausted, I like the evening clinic. We bring patients in quickly and spend more time with them. If a patient doesn't show up, we have a chance to catch up on the lab callbacks. Sometimes, we just sit and chat, catching up on each other's news. But tonight, there isn't a second to spare.

D. puts in the first evening patient, and I wait in the hall feeling a little bit sorry for myself. No desk, no privacy, twelve very long hours. I think of a nurse prac-titioner friend who works in a private office. She has a maple desk and her own nurse. When we talk, my friend asks, *how can you stand working in the clinic?*

It's true. Sometimes, in the clinic, hard work goes unrecognized. There isn't always respect all around, and there are a few providers who leave the difficult or foreign language–speaking patients to someone else. But when I see a nurse leading a dark-haired woman into an exam room, I know, without picking up the chart, that the woman is poor and alone in an unfamiliar country. No matter how trivial our encounter, no matter how little I actually do, she will thank me with sincerity and genuine gratitude. The patients I see are too often ignored, taunted, demeaned, unheard. Here, I can help them. So my answer to my friend is always the same. I like what I do.

6:00 P.M. In the next hour, I see three patients. The first is a woman with a new outbreak of herpes. She and I talk about the virus, about how it's transmitted. She wonders if her boyfriend was unfaithful. She asks if this virus will interfere with her ability to have children. Then she asks a question that takes my breath away: *Don't you see women all the time who are afraid?* Yes, I tell her. All the time.

Next is a woman with a long history of abnormal Paps, here for another one.

A pro at the various investigations and treatments, she sighs and crosses her fingers when I say the results will be back in about a week.

Then I see a teenager who thinks she may be pregnant and wants a test. *You don't have to call my mother, do you?* she asks. The test is negative.

7:00 P.M. When I open the next patient's chart, I remember her last visit a few weeks ago. When she'd first announced her pregnancy to her husband, he was furious. "Choose between me and the baby," he said. She chose the baby. Then, when I did her ultrasound, I'd found an "empty sac"—evidence that the pregnancy had failed. She wept so inconsolably that tears came to my own eyes. Her loss was double. Her husband was already gone, and now there would be no baby. Tonight, we discuss the results of her latest blood test. I tell her that the pregnancy hormone level in her body is back to normal. She can go on with her life.

More patients: a pregnant woman whose baby isn't moving. I send her upstairs to Labor and Delivery for monitoring. Another patient who, when L. walks in, asks if she could see me instead. L. comes out, red-faced, and practically throws the chart at me. Like all of us, she gets frazzled at the end of a twelve-hour shift. I know what it feels like when a patient looks you up and down and then announces they'd prefer someone else. This patient wants to talk, and so we do, although my tolerance is also wearing thin. I don't feel much like a saint about now.

7:45 P.M. We're finished with patients, so now I must slip from my nurse-skin back into my wife-skin. It's as if I have a whole day behind me and another whole day ahead. I help clean the rooms, enter labs into the computer, and lock up. We all clock out at 8:15 P.M.

I walk down the three flights of cement stairs to my car. It's dark, but I'm not afraid. A funny thing happens as I leave the clinic. I feel empty, and that space gets filled up with a nervous intolerance. If anyone tries to attack me now, he'll have to deal with a woman with a real short temper.

8:25 P.M. Home again. I resettle myself and do the things a woman does: sort the mail, check the answering machine, empty the dishwasher, throw in a wash load, figure out what to serve with leftover chicken.

8:57 P.M. Dinner. Chicken, peas, sweet potatoes mashed and buttered and tasting not bad at all. I'm beginning to relax when my husband says he could use a vacation. *Not me,* I say, teeth a little clenched. *I love working this hard.* "Cranky, aren't we?" he replies.

10:00 P.M. Propped up with pillows, I watch one hour of TV, the mindless hour I call it, the only way I can settle down enough to sleep. Tonight, it's an *ER* rerun.

11:00 P.M. My husband's a night owl. I fall asleep quickly and don't wake when he comes to bed. My last thought is to remember to ask the chief resident to schedule my patient's C-section and my other patient's induction, the one who came in for her first visit at forty-one weeks.

OCTOBER 8

2:00 A.M. I startle awake and open my eyes to the blue darkness. Did I forget anything? Did I make any mistakes? Was there anything I could have done better? Like shadows cast on a wavering screen, the faces of the patients I saw just hours ago float, mingle, and begin to fade. Today and the next day and the next, their faces will blend with the faces of other women, becoming the memories I carry with me.

First, Do No Harm

Milagros is an illegal alien, one of many who come to the women's clinic. She has a valid-looking social security card, but when we check, we find that four other patients claim the same number. Last month, she used the last name Lopez. This month, she signs in as "Milagros Hernandez." Then one of the nurses recognizes her. "Hey, Milagros," the nurse says in rapid-fire Spanish. "Make up your mind, *mi amor!* Pick one name and stick to it. You know we won't report you."

A few years ago, we saw few undocumented patients. Then, month by month, our census increased. Now, our appointment book holds only the names of women who've fled their homes in Ecuador, Colombia, Mexico, or Peru, leaving everything behind to follow husbands who are convinced life will be better in the United States. Here, a man can earn enough to send money home. Here, a pregnant woman can receive good medical care and have half a chance of delivering a healthy baby.

When the language barrier kept us from delivering good care, we hired Spanish-speaking secretaries and nurses. The residents and I learned Spanish on the job. Today, the TV is always tuned to the Spanish station, and patients chat in musical variations of their Ecuadorian, Puerto Rican, Dominican, or Chilean tongues. Inside our clinic, cultures merge, sometimes painfully, but our patients' illegal status isn't an issue we speak about.

Recently, Milagros was admitted to the hospital in her seventh month of pregnancy with out-of-control blood pressure. She's stable, but we can't discharge her.

Milagros has no permanent home. Shortly after she arrived in this country, she discovered she was pregnant. Her husband abandoned her. She sleeps on the floor of friends' apartments, moving every few days. She doesn't speak English and cannot read or write Spanish. We tried to treat her high blood pressure by asking Milagros to maintain bed rest, but her friends wouldn't let her lie on their floors all day. She can't return to Ecuador, nor does she want to. She wants her new baby to have what the three children she left behind don't have: food, medical care, shelter. Milagros has been in the maternity ward for three weeks, a hospitalization she can't afford.

If we discharge her, her blood pressure might become critical; then we'll have to deliver the baby prematurely. In that case, the neonatal intensive care unit will have to care for the baby, perhaps for months. If Milagros has no permanent address when the baby is ready for discharge, it will be placed in foster care.

At high-risk conference, we try to decide what to do about Milagros.

"We'd send any other patient home," the attending physician says.

"But," the chief resident says, "every time we discharge her, she goes back to work and her pressure hits the roof. If she doesn't work, she doesn't eat. Morally, how can we let her go?"

"Can't the visiting nurses help?" one of the medical students asks.

"Sure," the visiting nurse replies. "But whenever we try to find her, she's moved. If we call, no one answers. They think we're the authorities."

And so Milagros lingers. If her pressure cooperates, she'll probably deliver somewhere around her due date. If she finds a friend to volunteer an address and phone number, Milagros will leave with her baby. But "home" will still be a series of stopovers in already crowded apartments. Her only escape might be to find a new partner who will provide, at least temporarily, housing and food.

In a few years, she may learn enough English to take the bus or make an appointment without help. Because her baby will receive welfare, Milagros will have some money for rent and food. When her other children are grown, Milagros may send for them—if she's saved enough for their expensive, illegal, dangerous transport. For now, all she can do is pray that someday they'll be reunited; that this child, a U.S. citizen, might find a better life.

Before we admitted Milagros to the hospital, she always arrived in the clinic wearing the same skirt, the same shirt, the same thin sandals, even in winter. She survives at a level of poverty most North Americans can't imagine. Like most of the undocumented women we see, Milagros, if we allow it, will be a hard worker. But she will also be prone to injury and illness. Because she won't stay home if she is sick and because she'll ignore early warning signs of serious illness, she may continue to be an additional drain on our already overburdened health system.

I've heard the complaints: that soon the only language we'll hear in America is Spanish; that Latino immigrants deprive citizens of jobs; that those without any insurance—like Milagros—get everything for free. But the truth is, I don't know anyone who'd like to step into Milagros's life.

"Sort of like what my grandmother went through," my husband says when, after dinner, I tell him about Milagros. Newly arrived from a Russian shtetl, his grandmother spoke no English and, along with the Irish and Italians, was marginalized by more affluent immigrants. She raised five children; two became doctors. Two of her grandchildren became doctors. Today, those doctors take care of patients like Milagros.

During high-risk conference, I look around and see Dr. Clark, whose family surely came from the Irish slums. I see Elena, a brilliant resident who speaks Greek on the phone long distance to her family in Crete. I see Miriam, black-skinned African, whose ancestors arrived as slaves in the Caribbean. In the mirror, I see myself: the pale skin of my Scot ancestors, the coffee-brown hair of my Welsh great-grandfather (the troublemaker), the down-turned blue eyes of the Burt family, English trespassers on Native American soil who were carried off and sold to French missionaries in Canada during the French and Indian War.

I don't think Milagros should be turned out of the hospital. I can't imagine supporting the idea that she should be deported to Ecuador where she would once again exist in squalor. Assuming that we learn from history, I know that Milagros is, like our forebears, one of the new wave of Americans. I know that the bodegas and Spanish-only newspapers function as the Yiddish, Irish, and German markets and publications of early twentieth-century New York.

I don't know how we negotiate the years between the current influx of immigrant women and the future, when they will be the mothers and grandmothers of doctors and nurses whose skills will improve our country and who will, in turn, care for the next arrivals, whoever they may be. For now, I can only see Milagros, lying in her hospital bed, unable to communicate, with no one to call and no place to go. I can only imagine Milagros, walking out of the hospital with her baby, and I don't know how to help her.

Hearing the Stories behind
Our Patients' Words

It was September 11, 2001, and I was sitting at home in front of my computer revising the policies and procedures for the women's health clinic. Shortly after 9 A.M., my husband called from his office. "Turn on the TV," he said. "A plane just hit the World Trade Center." I turned on the TV exactly at the moment the second plane banked to knife into the glass and steel of Tower Two. As many of us did, I stood alternately crying or praying, unable to look away from the screen as the terrible events unfolded. The Pentagon was struck by a third plane. A fourth plane was detected, flying off course, and then it crashed in Shanksville, Pennsylvania, coring a fiery crater into a deserted field. Like a terrifying novel, the plot became more and more convoluted.

My first emotion, even before fear, was a diffuse, anguished compassion. I thought of the airline passengers who must have watched as the tower loomed before them. I thought about those people in the tower going about their early morning work routines, and about their families who, just hearing this news, would be frantic wondering if their loved ones were involved. Because I am a nurse, I thought of all the caregivers who rushed to the scene: paramedics, firefighters, policemen and women, doctors, nurses—anyone who thought they could help in any way.

Outside my window, it was a beautiful September day. There were birds at the feeder, yellow finches and downy woodpeckers. A young buck picked his way through our woods, a scene so peacefully oblivious that the contrast was bewildering. For seconds at a time, I could almost believe that what was happening on TV was a movie. Then, the towers collapsed, and with them, the naive belief that what happens to others could never happen to us.

I called my children because I wanted to hear their voices and know they were safe. My husband tried to phone his elderly mother, who lived eight blocks from the towers and would eventually be without electricity or water, unreachable for several days. As minutes passed, the broad and diffuse compassion that I'd felt at first became personal and individual. I began calling and emailing New York and Washington friends. Everything else became meaningless.

As the days went by, we learned exactly how much and how many had been lost, taught by the faces of the victims staring out at us from handmade posters and by the faces of their grieving families, by the faces of the rescue workers and those who stood applauding them, by the strained faces of our government officials and by the faces of the men and women in green scrubs waiting in the streets. Just as our patients become unexpectedly ill, just as thousands of men and women set out on their normal routines and were caught unaware, we became vulnerable.

In the wake of the events of September 11, I wondered how we would possibly go on. Just as we had to return to our lives in order to resist fear and terrorism, I decided to reinvest myself in the belief that patients' stories, victims' stories, can change our lives and help us to be better caregivers and better citizens. Certainly, in the days following, I learned how the *details* of individual lives can hone our feelings of compassion into a personal, focused, and active empathy.

At one point, I wondered what it would be like to be *there,* in the thick of it. What if I could be transported from my home in Connecticut, an hour away, and slip into the body of a woman in a Tower stairwell or a nurse waiting to receive victims in the ER, or a mother who'd left her home to stand waiting for news of her son? I wondered what it would *feel* like to be them. Listening to the tragic stories unfold in newspaper and news reports and hearing their families tell stories about their loved ones, we all could, in a metaphorical sense, suffer with them.

Maybe this is why the idea of "story" is so important to me. Because we nurses, who often come to our profession filled with that same amorphous compassion— that longing to help people—can, over time, lose sight of the *individual* patient and become numb to the particular kind of empathy that is difficult to sustain and yet essential to the delivery of excellent health care. It isn't easy to go from bedside to bedside or to muster the emotional response that enables us to best serve each patient. We may also mistake the pleasure and relief we feel at our own response to human suffering, or the pride we feel at our own technical expertise, for genuine caring.

We see patients suspended at atypical moments in their lives, often knowing them only from the external information they present—symptoms, test results, chief complaints, and physical findings. Just as I couldn't actually enter into the bodies of the 9/11 victims or their families to feel what it was like to be them, none of us can truly become our patients or experience their suffering. But stories of caregiving—patients' stories, nurses' stories, doctors' stories—can help us to sharpen our empathic skills, enabling us to be better, more humane and even more emotionally fulfilled providers.

When, for the first time, we stand in our student uniforms at the bedside of a suffering patient, what we feel is often anxiety and a formless but intense emotion based not only on the patient's situation but also on our own. Maybe we recall the sorrow we'd felt when someone close to us died, or we identify with what it was like when we were ill or alone. As students, we vow we will never forget the small details, images that distress and move us yet also serve to make a patient's suffering tangible: an old woman's blue nightgown, the worn slipper peeking out from under a bed, a child's book closed on the nightstand. We promise ourselves *we* will never become coolly clinical or distanced, as it seems some of our teachers are. We believe that, as nurses, we will *always* be above pettiness, anger, fatigue, and alienation.

When I became a student nurse, I felt that way. Then, slowly, something happened. I learned a new language made up of concrete clinical terms about illness and cure, a language that was musical but opaque, one that identified me as part of an elite group and so separated me from my patients. Memorizing facts and figures that often had little relationship to any *specific* patient, I lost sight of the individual: that woman in the blue nightgown and that particular child whose book was forgotten on the bedside stand. Instead I became fascinated with diseases. I looked forward to each unusual case, to each odd clinical finding that the attending doctors labeled "fascinomas." Like the residents around me, I liked the challenge of taking care of complex, critically ill patients. And, like medical students who can only dissect their cadaver if they cover the body's face, I didn't allow myself to become involved. In order to do what we had to do, sometimes we chose to believe that what *we* knew about a patient, suspended at the moment of his or her illness, was the only version of the story we needed.

What jolted me out of that clinical distance and commanded that I pay attention to each patient's unique story? I don't know—maybe it was my years on the oncology ward; maybe it was because as I sat with dying patients I became more aware of my own mortality. Most likely it was the poetry I wrote about my work, the heightened, sensual, and metaphorical words on the page that blasted apart that learned, impersonal medical language and gave me back the surprise and emotional urgency that accompanies a student's first glimpse of another's suffering. A few years after I'd graduated from nursing school, patients had become that unknowable other world, the one that I had learned to keep at arm's length in order to survive. Poetry changed that.

· · ·

What is it that happens to us as we travel the path from student to seasoned practitioner? How is it that we sometimes feel so fragile that if we stop to confront suffering, we believe we ourselves might shatter? How is it that if a patient or their family dares to ask us for *one more thing,* we can close up and wave them away?

Well, we might respond, *we know how that happens:* too many diseases, too much to learn, too much to read, failures that seem to outnumber successes, petty demands, managed care, loss of control, numbing routine, false pride, ungrieved personal tragedy, fear of lawsuits, inability to make decisions based on patients' desires, too much paperwork, the command from administration to avoid overtime, and on and on. We might ask each other, especially in the wake of 9/11, of Hurricane Katrina, of the war in Iraq, how does anyone hold on to the human underbelly of caring without becoming numb? How do we enable students to discover the measure of empathy that will connect them to, rather than alienate them from, their patients?

Maybe one answer is that we can try to teach them that each patient, each nurse, each physician, each family member, each volunteer or orderly or tech— anyone in any way involved with a patient's illness—has a story. Maybe we can ask students to seek out and pay attention to those stories, both those on the page and those they hear around them every day on the wards, in the elevators, and in the cafeteria. Maybe every student has his or her *particular* patient, one whose story splits open the world, enabling that student to see and feel both the uniqueness and the oneness of all suffering.

If we caregivers can write, talk, or read about our experiences with patients, those stories might transform us, reaffirm us, and give us the energy we need to reach out to our patients again and again. Patients' stories are more than their clinical case histories. Patients' lives, like our own, are rich, thick, complicated, shifting, multilayered, and rambling. Reading about patients and caregivers gives students, as well as experienced practitioners, emotional templates that help to foster and maintain empathic and ethical responses to actual patients.

Stories also offer us solace, the ability to move out of "clinical time" and into "creative" or "literary" time. Think of a code 99 or of the first moments of the terrorist attack. Clinical time is gone in a finger snap, unalterable, and embedded in fact. Clinical time can be stressful and filled with fear, shame, and guilt, perhaps particularly for students. It's a time for quick decisions made with little reflection. Thankfully, it can also be a time of success and poignant intimacy.

In contrast, creative time is open-ended. In it, we can analyze or alter the ending. Here, our concern is not only about what is factually true but also about what is emotionally true. A story or poem can suggest the depth and breadth of a patient's life; stories or poems give us time to discover and reframe our emotional responses.

Creative time allows for reassessment, replaying, and rejoicing. It gives us the opportunity to heal, to learn how we might better react next time, and also to bond in celebration. Stories and poems, whether we write them or read them, teach us to walk gently alongside illness, despair, and recovery. My own impetus to write about my interactions with patients, and to encourage other caregivers to write about theirs, is personal rather than academic. There is a thin line between a nurse and her patient—perhaps only a day or a phone call between comfort and poverty, between health and disease. I believe that we become wiser, kinder individuals when we share another's suffering and recovery. I believe that our own lives become clearer and take on new shape when we listen to another's story, especially if we can recognize that we, like our patients or the victims of any tragedy—such as September 11, 2001, or the Indian Ocean tsunami that swept so many away in 2004, or the hurricane, eight months later, that forever changed the lives of those in New Orleans, or the war in Iraq that seems to go on and on, taking so many lives with it—are embodied beings who struggle from day to day.

If we write about what we experience—even the simplest poems or stories will do—we are truly paying attention. Such careful consideration, both in the flesh and on the page, might enable us to offer our hearts and thereby become wiser, kinder health care providers.

Body Teaching

Last summer, two of the new interns who joined our team in the women's health clinic were men; otherwise, all our care providers are female. Because our clinic is located in a teaching hospital, there's also a stream of students passing through regularly. Medical residents spend a mandatory week or two with us, usually grudgingly, to sharpen their pelvic exam skills, and nervous medical students in short white coats do six-week rotations. About 60 percent of these students are male. They plan to become orthopods, pediatricians, or internists—rarely do they want to pursue OB-GYN. They say it's becoming a female-dominated field. If, after his weeks with us, a student does say he might consider OB-GYN, he usually says it's because he likes the combination of surgery and medicine.

Well-versed in syndromes and lab values and auscultation of the heart, these students come to our clinic and find themselves suddenly disoriented. Here, they can't hide behind shifting sodium values or unstable hemoglobins. In our world, a student must touch a woman's breasts and probe her vagina. He must learn to delineate the uterus, invisible beneath a woman's skin, and he must perfect the maneuvers that cause her ovaries to slip between his examining hands. Here, he must come face to face with the flesh and all its implications: fecundity and longing, sexuality and pain. Here, his fingertips must become as sensitive as a safecracker's.

The choice, the entire rotation, seems more natural for our female students. Although they can be just as anxious about performing their first pelvic exams, they've often had Pap tests and internals themselves. It's easier to teach them; they share an intuitive common world with our patients and enjoy caring for other women. But I'd rather teach the men. They're the ones who are most uncomfortable and who must acquire a facility that goes beyond the mere perfection of the exam. Teaching them, I try to use the insights that arise from my multiple roles—I'm a woman who has also been a patient, a nurse as well as a nurse practitioner. I'm keenly aware that I am a woman teaching a man and, in a role reversal even more volatile, a nurse teaching a doctor whose authority will be, ultimately, more respected than mine. Most of all, I am a female guide who must step out of her body, casting off any suggestions of sensuality or privilege, when it is precisely my body that allows me to excel at teaching this intimate exam.

"Come with me," I say to this month's medical student. I'll call him Raymond, a tall, quiet third-year from a big university program. When I ask, he tells me that he thinks he wants to be an oncologist, but he's not sure yet. We go down the hall and stand for a moment outside room three, where our patient—I'll call her Maria Lopez—waits for us. Raymond tells me he's done several pelvic exams before. Nevertheless, he confesses, he's never quite sure what he's *feeling*. I catch hold of his inadvertent double entendre and think perhaps we're going to have a real conversation, one that addresses the multilevel aspects of the exam we're about to perform: what he's feeling in his doctor's body, both physically and emotionally; what the patient is feeling; and how, as I stand by observing, my body responds, remembering. Then Raymond clarifies. "I can never tell if the uterus is retroverted or anteverted," he says.

Before we knock on the exam room door, I encourage him.

"Don't worry," I say. "The exam takes practice. It's more important that you listen to Maria and watch her face. Let her give you clues to what *she* is feeling."

Maria, who has been a clinic patient for years, sits uneasily at the end of the exam table. She has delivered three babies with us and lost one with us too, a spontaneous abortion that occurred a month ago. Today our job is to make sure everything has returned to normal. We have to palpate her uterus to make sure it's firm and small again after the early miscarriage of her pregnancy. We have to ask her about bleeding and the resumption of intercourse. Most essential, we have to inquire about Maria's grief and healing, those extraordinary processes that trail along behind a woman's life like silk scarves.

Raymond, who I introduce to Maria as *un estudiante,* will conduct the exam. I, in my long flowered skirt and my woman's body, will observe. My own breasts have heft and weight, and, when he palpates Maria's breasts, I will know how to direct him, resisting the urge to move his hands aside and show him. When he attempts the pelvic exam, I am aware of my own body, its strength and its fragility. Surely this happens to Raymond when he examines other men. He recognizes their body signals and is more careful, because at some level the borders of his body and the patient's body meld. I step back and prepare to assist him.

I can never be sure how Raymond or any student will come to terms with what he's thinking or feeling when he examines a patient. Like many students on their way to more desired rotations, Raymond might simply breeze through the clinic, unaffected. I might teach him to identify the size of the uterus (a peach, a lemon, a grapefruit), how to twirl the Pap spatula deftly around a patient's cervical Os, and how to perform a thorough breast exam, but my goal is also to teach him what physical and emotional responses these maneuvers elicit in his female patients. As Raymond begins to examine Maria, I tell him that because I am a woman, I'm privileged to have some idea of what another woman experiences during an exam. Even so, I add, no one can ever truly know what someone else is feeling.

But there is another way of knowing. I can *imagine* how Maria might feel, torn between shame and fear as Raymond steps forward to examine her body. I suspect that today she thinks her body has turned against her, expelling her fetus, a baby she very much desired. Yet, like any woman, she cannot escape her body's whims. Tingling breasts and monthly blood flow, hormonal flushes and roller coaster dizziness, fertile pregnancies and even lost babies are a part of our lot. If Raymond can understand this—if he watches Maria's face and notes how her legs relax or tense, if her vaginal introitus contracts in surprise at his touch or loosens around the speculum, if she moves away from his hands or accepts them—then he too might come to know Maria and help her make peace with her body.

I can project my own experiences as a female patient onto my encounters with others. Maria's intimate parts, like those of all women, are private. In order to remain healthy, we must permit trespass, lie on our backs as Maria does now, letting her knees fall open, relaxing her thighs and her buttocks. Surely Raymond too has been exposed and examined, vulnerable and afraid.

He inserts the metal speculum. "Aim down," I tell him. My memory of how this feels is vivid. "Be careful to avoid the urethra."

Maria looks at the ceiling as Raymond peers through the speculum's blades to find her cervix and examine it, as he removes the speculum, as he fumbles (now he fumbles, but soon he will perform this gesture as easily and unconsciously as he walks) to reach his lubricated, gloved fingers to the very cul-de-sac of Maria's vagina. She gives the slightest wince, and Raymond begins to sweat. I reach for Maria's hand. He has hurt her. Tiny drops of moisture spring from the hair follicles on his upper lip.

"This is an uncomfortable exam," I tell him, "and it's important that you're thorough. But remember, she can't see what you're doing. Explain what you're going to do before you do it. Talk to her, and she might be more comfortable." Maria and I exchange glances and roll our eyes. *Eso nos pasa,* I say to her, *por ser mujer.* This is what we women must endure. I keep hold of her hand.

Turning to Raymond, I explain the basic uterine positions: anteverted, retroverted, or midplane. Maria's uterus, I know from her previous visits, is retroflexed, retroverted to the maximal degree. I tell Raymond that when a woman's uterus is retroflexed, it can cause perpetual distress: pain with intercourse as the penis nudges the cervix and jostles the uterus; difficult exams, as often the retroflexed uterus can only be adequately palpated with an uncomfortable recto-vaginal investigation. I repeat this in Spanish and Maria nods in agreement.

"Identify the thin wall between rectum and vagina. Locate the firm uterine fundus flexed back under the cervix, a bulge that impinges on the rectal canal," I say.

"Wow," Raymond says, beaming. "I think I got it."

He leans into this exam, steadying his right hand, the one that has luckily found the uterus. Maria has turned her face to the wall, but Raymond doesn't notice. Not that he is callous or mechanical. He's preoccupied. First he had to deal with his fear of awkwardness, of hurting his patient. Now he's simply elated that he has succeeded in mastering one more thing in the chain of a thousand things that he must learn. He isn't aware of Maria's embarrassment. No, it's more accurate to say that he doesn't *feel* Maria's embarrassment. Later, I will ask him if he recalls Maria's turned-away stare, her silent endurance. "Think of how invaded she must have felt," I'll say.

When the exam is over (I have to check as well to be sure that her uterus is normal and her ovaries free of cysts), Raymond stands back, as if he no longer dare touch her, while I help Maria sit up. It will take Maria's body an hour or so to recover. Her uterus will be slightly sore, rattled. Her ovaries will ache. The lubricant will irritate her vagina. Later, a gelatinous glob of it may slip out of her at an inconvenient moment. Her relationship with Raymond will remain a wild contradiction. He is a man and a stranger. He has *seen* her.

I think he too must be lost in a whirl of emotions: pride at his skill; exhilaration at his increasing clinical familiarity with the female body; maybe even an innocent pleasure at the *otherness* of its mystery and velvety passageway, the firmness of the womb, the contrast (unconscious or realized) between this unerotic exam and the lovemaking he shares with his wife. I imagine that he feels ill at ease as well, both indebted to Maria and detached from her—grateful that she has let him practice on her body and yet about to forget her.

After we tell Maria how sorry we are that her pregnancy has miscarried and after she has wept on my shoulder, Raymond and I bid her good-bye. We walk back to the residents' lounge where he writes the details of this encounter in Maria's chart. As we sit together, Raymond seems to recognize (as if by revelation) that he simply can't include Maria's version of their transaction. In that instant, he transcends the mechanical and acknowledges the personal. What he writes in Maria's chart, he realizes, is only *his* side of the story; and so he must pay close attention to any hints that he might gather, like Hansel and Gretel's bread crumbs, that will help him expand his vision. If Raymond can recall his most human moments and translate those memories into a shared vulnerability with his patients, he might yet master that elusive *knowing.*

"Thanks for your help," he says. "I guess you've been there."

I agree, and he struggles to find a way to ask me. "What's it like for the patient? What was it like for Maria—what is that exam like from a woman's point of view?"

I hesitate, not sure of where to begin or how much I might personally have to reveal, but Raymond leans toward me, interested and fully engaged. I'm touched by his question, heartened by his sensitivity. He puts down his pen, pushes aside his red manual of gynecological facts, for now abandoning his desire to identify uterine orientation or cystic ovaries. He wants to step into his patient's body and know what *she* is feeling. He wants to know how this exam is experienced, and that will help him to understand the subtext of women's health. He's asking me to lead him by memory, by my own body's recollection, as if I might go on ahead, mapping out the path that he must follow by faith alone. I tell Raymond that he just might become a wonderful doctor.

As we talk, finding language to soar above the level of rote skill, I realize that I'm not simply teaching Raymond and the other male students how to do a proficient pelvic exam. I'm teaching them my body.

Tattoos

Alex comes into the back room and closes the door. "I can't believe it," he says. "You should see this girl."

We look up from our charts. Alex's face is splotchy and he looks very young.

"What?" Linda asks. Alex is in his first year of OB-GYN residency—not exactly brand-new but not very experienced either. Next year he'll blossom, suddenly becoming more self-confident and realizing how much he's learned. Linda, a third-year resident, and I glance at each other. I've been a nurse practitioner in the clinic for sixteen years now; I've seen lots of residents pass through. Nothing they say surprises me.

"She has the greatest tattoo I've ever seen. I wish I had a camera."

Oh, I think.

I guess this is a revelation for Alex. The women who come into our clinic like to decorate, and sometimes all they have to adorn—all they have to call their own—are their bodies. I remember the first time I saw a patient splendid in her verdant green and bright blue tattoos. When I lifted the drape to begin her exam, I had to stifle a gasp.

A bird of paradise twined around the curve of her right arm, blue and green feathers flowed over her elbow. There were tropical flowers of every color and variety imaginable growing from her shoulder to her breasts, cascading over the slope of them, circling the nipples which alone had been spared and, in contrast, appeared to be pale, less exotic buds. Animals roamed across her belly—a zebra with black and white whorls along its back and a tail that spread coarse black hairs over her hip, and a lioness with yellow eyes. On her left arm were a series of incomplete black line drawings longing for color.

"My boyfriend won't tattoo me when I'm pregnant," she'd explained.

I was doing what good health professionals are not supposed to do. I was surveying the length and breadth of her, painted and etched like a canvas. When she lifted her heels into the stirrups and slid down to the end of the table for her exam, she was a ripple of color, gliding like a snake. A forest of vines inched down her thighs; here and there oranges and apples waited to be plucked. These were not the homemade tattoos some patients have, ugly blue scars from a novice's needle wrapped in thread, stuck in a cork, and dipped in ink. These were beautiful, dreamlike images. Amazing.

I told her so.

"Yeah," she replied. "He's an artist and he thinks I'm a piece of paper."

I tried to concentrate on her exam. Every time she moved, her skin glowed and the tattooed images temporarily distorted, as if she were a living LCD monitor touched with a fingertip.

When her exam was over, she put on her T-shirt and a pair of jeans carefully ripped to expose the eyes of the lioness. Not just another poor white girl from downtown, this lady was one of a kind. The way she walked, holding her head up, I could see she knew it.

"Those tattoos are something, aren't they?" I smile at Alex who's still shaking his head as he sits down to write in the patient's chart. Then, egging each other on, the residents make a list.

"Remember Tinker Bell tattooed on that pregnant patient's belly?" asks Rick, another third-year resident. Linda says, "Yeah, and when she was in her eighth month how Tinker Bell looked like some misshapen monster?" I can picture the tattoo—one wing flapped like a blighted arm and the other was rippled with stretch marks—but I can't place the patient's face.

Linda recalls one young patient who looked demure and shy but who nonetheless displayed, right below her umbilicus, a bloated heart with a dagger piercing it. Three drops of blood hung from the tattooed blade, a girl-gang insignia. Rick counters with "Did you ever see that one of a pair of snake eyes dice?" And there are so many patients with geometric, intricately tattooed bracelets and anklets that we could never number them all. Roses on shoulders and hearts over the breasts are a dime a dozen.

I like whispering with the residents about these intimate details that we are supposed to see but certainly not discuss. "Let's face it," we've said to each other. "Some of our patients are fascinating." When patients come in moist and steamy in the summer and peel off their clothes to reveal the secret flowers and humming birds, insects and hearts forever bound to their bodies, it's all we can do to resist staring at those washes of color, the small scrolls and loops that bead the white, black, tan, or yellow skin of these cheeky, decorated, in-your-face girls.

Often enough, there's ugliness instead of beauty. One day I examined a high school girl who sported a badly drawn rose on her arm. It was an amateur job, the ink lines wide and wavering, the color more rust than rose vermilion. We talked about the transmission of hepatitis and HIV, about prevention and testing.

Then there are the patients whose tattoos are sinister. Not feisty, not proud, those women are objectified, terrifyingly marked. I wonder how they'll look when they're eighty, their crinkled skin enfolding the skulls etched onto their abdomens. When I examine them, I flinch from touching the symbols and images carved into their skin.

Around me, the residents are laughing, tears running down their cheeks. Most of them are so chronically overtired it doesn't take much to set them off, and now Alex has jumped up to snap imaginary pictures—a forbidden photo shoot. He says he loves the tattooed lady, and we tease him about finding a woman of his own. The discussion disintegrates.

They must be extra stressed, like surgeons who joke in the midst of open-heart surgery just to tether themselves to the earth and still their trembling hands. They're saying what they'd never reveal to anyone—how every day we see the most astonishing variety of sights, intimacies normally hidden from public view. We see what mothers or lovers see, that which is reflected only in the private gaze or the bedroom mirror: beautiful patients and plain patients; fascinating body piercings and horrible scars; tattoos that make us smile or give us chills.

I almost describe, but don't, the kind of body markings I remember from my days and nights in intensive care and the oncology ward: ulcerations bubbling with pus, cleaned every shift by nurses who never grimaced, never turned away; charred flesh that turned black and putrid; deep sutured incisions that split open, spilling out pink intestines against the stark white gauze. I don't remember nurses or doctors talking or joking about these sights. I think we knew, instinctively, that any patient's wound might some day be our own.

Linda gets up and huffs out of the room. "Okay," she says. "This has gone too far." She thinks we've come too close to our patients' bodies. Perhaps we've really come too close to our own issues of exposure and restraint, even to our own fears. One of the nurses, curious, comes in with a chart in her hand. She leans against the wall, listening. I concentrate on the open book in front of me.

I suppose that talking about what we see lets us maintain a safe, necessary line, that very thin boundary between "us" and "them" that we hesitate to step over. Perhaps such backroom banter defuses the erotic possibilities. It allows us to help our patients without imposing our own standards or practices and without judging theirs. This impartiality lets our patients stay in control, and for many of them, taking charge of their bodies is the only way they can take possession of their lives. Without money and often without adequate education, our patients might not have much hope about their futures or their children's futures. But some have friends with steady hands and an uncanny talent with needle and ink.

Maybe our fascination comes from envy. Our clinic patients are free to ornament themselves as they wish—to be a little wild—while we clinicians are restricted to stark clothing, small earrings, not-too-long hair, and somber voices.

Truth is, the *particular* bodies we see fade from our memories almost as quickly as our patients walk out the door. While we might recall a particularly exotic tattoo or a devastating injury, the details of an individual patient's nakedness vanish—the images soon dissolve into a wavering fog of light and color. In the back room, we may laugh, but our laughter is wary. After all, we doctors and nurses are patients too, guardians of our own body secrets. We are also scanned and probed; perhaps we each have some little oddity that, we trust, remains only in our examiner's inner eye.

Alex's beeper sounds, and he is summoned to the emergency room. Linda comes back into the room and announces that she's due in the OR. Rick waves and says he has to do an ultrasound on a woman pregnant with twins. The nurse hands me the chart and says, "Looks like you're the only one left to see this patient." I nod. The residents and I button up our white coats and hurry to do as we're told.

Breaking Bad News

I'm just about to flip open the patient's chart to find out why she is here when I see a note stuck on the front of the folder. "Positive for chlamydia," is scribbled in the secretary's handwriting. "Here for treatment."

I'm tempted to let one of the residents deal with this patient—but it's high-risk pregnancy day and we're sure to get backed up. Anyway, I've been a nurse for years. Giving bad news is part of my job.

Reviewing the chart, I read that the patient, Ellen, is in the fourteenth week of her first pregnancy. Three days ago, she'd experienced burning with urination and vague pelvic pain. She'd come to the clinic, terrified that something was wrong with her pregnancy. The resident who saw her collected a urine culture to make sure Ellen didn't have an infection and did a pelvic exam, checking for simple infections, like yeast, and culturing for more serious infections. Yesterday the nurse called and left a message on Ellen's phone: *Come into the clinic tomorrow. We have your test results.* Looking at the chart, I find that everything came back negative except the cervical culture. Ellen has chlamydia, a sexually transmitted disease, and I'm the one who must tell her.

Giving bad news to patients is a special talent, something no amount of education can teach. When I was in nursing school and, later, in nurse practitioner training, there were no courses called "How to tell a patient she has cancer," "How to tell a father his child has died," or "How to tell a pregnant woman she has a sexually transmitted disease." Breaking bad news is an on-the-job skill learned only in the doing, in the holding of patients' hands, and in the simple comforting acts that suddenly erase the distance between nurse and patient: the hug that keeps someone on her feet; the way we sometimes let patients see the tears in our own eyes.

In Intensive Care, I learned to deliver bits of stunning information as if they were updates from some distant, unfamiliar city. Calling a newly admitted child's parent, I'd say, "Your son's been admitted to ICU." Then, I'd wait a few seconds for the implication in my voice to travel the phone wires. On the cancer ward, I perfected the arts of acknowledging the approach of death and staying with patients until death arrived. I'd grip a woman by the shoulders, look into her face. "I was with your husband when he died," I'd say. "He didn't go alone."

When I came to the women's clinic, I thought joy would outweigh tragedy. Mostly, that's true. But bad news here is particularly difficult to hear—it often involves new life, and it can pierce the soul. I've told mothers that their pregnancies won't survive. I've announced that my fingers have palpated the solitary breast nodule that could be cancer. More and more often, I have to tell young women that their bodies are infected with diseases they get only from making love. How, I wonder, will Ellen react to the news that she has chlamydia?

Some women nod and smile, unable to comprehend how they, who are faithful to their partners, could have a sexually transmitted disease. They look at me with such innocent bewilderment that I'm afraid for them. Then, when they finally understand, they weep or become so angry that even the bland, beige clinic walls seem unable to contain their fury.

Other women blush and lower their eyes. They have secrets to tell, and sometimes they do: a brief affair; a man who, they thought, loved them. These women are dazed. They thought they were only following their hearts. When I say, "You'll have to notify *all* your partners," they feel abandoned. "How can I tell my husband?" they ask, or, "How can I tell my boyfriend?" I never have the right answer.

Most often, patients receiving bad news crumble before me. Their skin blanches. They lose their breath, as if punched in the stomach. It's difficult to watch their suffering.

I've found it's best to give bad news over time, bit by bit, like you'd give a child small bites of food that are easier to swallow. Patients can only take in what they're ready to accept. Of course, bad news must be followed by a list of options, as if those might be the sips of water that help soothe the lump in the throat. We sometimes think that if we can offer patients other tests, specialists to see, the possibility of cure, then we can also give them hope. After so many years in health care, I've learned that all we can really give our patients is what we would want for ourselves. We can listen. We can accept that we are, after all, *like* our patients, vulnerable and afraid.

I take the chart and go into room 4, where Ellen sits on the exam table. A man—I assume it's her husband—waits beside her on a chair. *Oh boy,* I think to myself. *This will be twice as hard.*

"Hi Ellen. I'm Cortney, a nurse practitioner here in the clinic." I extend my hand to her and then face the man. "Hi," I say. "And you are. . . ?"

"Max," he answers.

"I got a message about test results," Ellen explains. "Is everything okay?" She rests one hand on her belly.

This exact moment—the uncertainty and possibility contained in the pause before I answer—is one of the things I dislike most about delivering bad news, perhaps because I never plan what to say ahead of time but wait until I can evaluate a patient's emotional reserve and then intuit how to proceed. Straightforward? With a maternal hug? Offhand and casual?

During this pause, I also feel guilty, as if I'm not simply a messenger but also somehow responsible for a patient's soon-to-be-visible anguish. I've learned that words are like stones. Tossed into the vast expanse of a patient's life, their impact causes shock waves. In ever-widening circles, everyone is affected. What was to be a patient's future is wrenched into a different shape and becomes, eventually, the past she'd like to forget. Sometimes, patients forever associate us with the information we've delivered. I don't want to cause pain. Like any nurse or doctor, I want patients to like me.

A physician once told me that he "soft-pedals" the news, making a dire situation sound not so awful. He wants to spare patients pain, but I think evasiveness leads to misunderstanding. I can't skirt the issues to avoid hurting a patient's feelings. At the same time, I know what it's like to have everything changed by a single test result or one damning word.

Ellen, even before I speak, looks hollow, as if the smallest blow could shatter her. Max looks anxious. I picture them raising their individual shields against anything that might alter their world.

"Ellen, I have your cervical culture results. Do you want Max to be here when we discuss them?"

I sit down by the exam table so I'm close to Ellen. After all, *she* is my patient. Part of me wants to say, "You might want to hear this alone." But there's another side of me, one I don't like, that wants to say, *let him stay. Let him be devastated too.*

"Yes, he can stay," she says.

I've never met Ellen before, a common occurrence in the clinic. In some ways, I'm glad. Being the messenger can be more difficult when I have a long-term relationship with a patient I've come to care about. In other ways, sometimes it's easier to give bad news when I've treated a patient over time. Then when I arrive with disastrous results in hand, she knows I'll support her, that her misfortune will become our common grief.

"Ellen, your culture came back positive for an infection called chlamydia."

"Oh, God. Is that something that could hurt the baby?"

"Not if it's treated, and we've caught it in time. After we talk, I'll give you an antibiotic to take. And Max?" I turn to him. "You'll have to see your doctor and get treated too. It's important that you refrain from intercourse until you've both taken medication."

Max opens and closes his hands. I notice he's not wearing a wedding ring.

"I don't understand," Ellen says. "How did I get this?"

"Chlamydia is a sexually transmitted disease. You get it from having sex with someone who has it."

"But I'm only with my husband."

"You get this infection when you have intercourse with someone who is already infected."

If I have to, I'll say this over and over. Bad news has to be given in short, strong sentences; otherwise, it's impossible to hear. Even when it involves the simplest absolutes—he's dying, she has cancer—bad news takes time to understand. I see Ellen struggling. If she only has sex with Max, she caught this infection from him. If she has sex with other men, this could have come from any of them. Once a man or woman has this infection, they can spread it to every partner they have.

The room is uncomfortably quiet. My pulse quickens. I want to make every-thing better. I could say, *it's very common—more than 4 million cases of chlamydia occur annually in the U.S.,* but that would be soft-pedaling, turning the attention away from Ellen's individual dilemma.

"I only have sex with Max." She looks at me as if I might shelter her from the image that, like a sudden eclipse, has darkened her imagination.

I place my hand on Ellen's knee. Tears fill her eyes and she purses her lips. When she goes to wipe her cheek, she begins to sob. I stand and put one arm around her, mindful of the newness of our relationship and the ambiguity of my role. I bring both the poison and the cure.

Max says, "I don't have any symptoms. I couldn't have given her anything."

"This infection might not cause any symptoms. That's why it's so difficult to detect."

"This means Max got it from someone and gave it to me?" Ellen's face is blotchy.

"I don't know, Ellen. Chlamydia can be dormant in the body for months."

"We've been together three years," she says.

"Married for one," Max adds.

Ellen turns on him. "Does that mean you've only been faithful to me for one?"

I don't interrupt.

"Tests can be wrong," Max says. He paces beside Ellen, who now holds both hands on her not-yet-enlarged belly, as if to cradle her fetus.

I say, "Although it is possible to have a false positive result, the type of test we use is rarely inaccurate."

I'm accustomed to this back and forth rapid firing of questions. Such a debate always occurs as patients sort and assimilate the facts that accompany bad news. How did it happen? When did it happen? Are you sure? The one question that I can never, ever answer is *why did this happen?* Patients think bad news might be easier to accept if only it came with some reason, some lesson, or someone to blame.

"We're having a baby," she says, half to me and half to Max. "How could you do this?"

"I didn't do anything," he says. "I could never do anything like that, and you know it."

I try to read his anger, then hers. If I could ignore her embarrassment and his indignation, I might suppose they were the perfect couple. I never know which patients will someday become the recipients of bad news. You can't tell just by looking.

"I recently spoke to another couple with the same problem," I say. "They decided to trust each other, take their antibiotics, and move on. We have to treat this infection. I know it's not as easy to heal the emotional effects."

In the grand list of bad news, some items are worse than others. I feel better when I can convince myself that bad news might also be the beginning of recovery, as I hope it will be for Ellen and Max. But in the end, grief is grief. It doesn't come neatly measured, and we can't compare one pain to another. There's nothing to be gained by telling a patient, "It could be worse." For Ellen and Max right now, this is grief enough.

I give Ellen four antibiotic tablets and watch as she takes them. I hand her a pamphlet about chlamydia. Max asks, "Can't you treat me too?" and I tell him that this is a women's clinic. We don't treat men. I give him the number of the STD clinic where he can be treated for free. He accepts this information but tips his head as if he hears something behind my words. Later, I'll replay our conversation. After all, I'm still trying to learn this technique, the best way to give bad news. Do I take sides? Even when I try not to, do I sometimes point a silent finger? Later, I'll wish I had a neat formula to follow. Then I'll think, *no.* Only we humans give and receive bad news. It must remain, therefore, a messy and imperfect skill.

In this case, I'll never know if the chlamydia test was falsely positive, if Ellen had another partner, or if it was Max who'd had a fling. One thing I know about bad news is that it comes out of nowhere. Once it arrives, it never really goes away.

I shake their hands and say I hope I'll see them again. I ask Ellen to call me if she wants to talk or has any questions. When they walk out of the exam room and down the hall, Max takes Ellen's arm. She doesn't draw away.

We caregivers sometimes have allies when we give bad news—patients find information on the Internet, and there are support groups for almost every ailment. Nevertheless, the initial announcement of bad news is always a solitary event, shared by patient and caregiver. When I'm the caregiver, all I can do is try to bring kindness, as well as truth, to the encounter: a hand's brief pressure, a silent standing by—anything that might help steady the heart.

Becoming Flora

She was the last patient to arrive that August Friday, an urgent add-on at the end of the day. The secretary's note, a terse fragment, oozed condemnation—"Patient 22-weeks pregnant, thinks her water broke a few nights ago but didn't bother to call"—an attitude I was all too ready to pick up and run with. It had been a long busy week, and I was tired. Tired of standing, tired of listening, tired of doing exams, tired of the noisy kids in the waiting room, and tired of pleading with those mothers who continued to smoke, drink, do drugs, or jeopardize their pregnancies in other ways.

I took a deep breath and closed my eyes for a second. Then I walked down the hall and knocked on the door of exam room three.

The woman (I'll call her Flora) sat at the end of the exam table, undressed and draped from the waist down—blond, angular, jittery, and nail bitten. I wondered if she was high. I stood over her, fully dressed and crisp in my white lab coat. My smile was automatic and superficial.

"Hello Flora," I said. "I understand you think your water might have broken. Tell me what happened."

"I *know* my water broke," she said. "I mean it was like a *flood* or something. It was maybe a day or two ago. I don't know, maybe last weekend? I can't remember."

I moved the rolling stool closer to the table and sat down. Flora's legs were thin and rashy. Her feet were bare, half moons of dirt were under the toenails, and thick yellow calluses hardened her soles. I remember thinking that those calluses might be an apt metaphor for Flora's life.

"Is the baby moving?" I asked.

"I guess," she said. "Maybe not so much today."

"Are you having contractions?"

Flora shrugged and scratched her nose with her index finger. She had tattoos on her knuckles, the do-it-yourself kind made with a cork, a needle, and some blue ink. One tattoo was a heart with an arrow through it. The other was a heart torn in two, its jagged edges no longer approximated. She caught me staring.

"Oh these. I did some time in Hanover," she explained, referring to a women's prison a few hours away.

"Broken hearts," I said, feeling a glimmer of empathy. "I guess we've all been there."

"No shit," Flora said, laughing and throwing her head back. I could see her teeth, small and uneven but brilliantly white. She was almost pretty. When I pulled the stirrups out of the exam table and motioned her into position, she apologized for her unshaven legs. I placed the sterile speculum into her vagina and a pool of foul, greenish amniotic fluid spilled down the speculum handle.

"Uh oh," I said, looking over the sheet to see her face. "Your water has definitely broken. And I think you've got an infection. What's been going on?" In my mind's eye I pictured her at an all-night party. I conjured her man, his grimy fingers. I began to feel remarkably clean, conveniently forgetting the seamier details of my own past.

After finishing the exam, I pushed back from the table, dropped the speculum into a bucket of disinfectant, and stripped off my gloves. My fingers were moist and wrinkled. My gold wedding band sparkled under the exam light.

"We'll have to get you right up to Labor and Delivery," I said. "It looks like your water's been ruptured for a few days—"

"Good," she interrupted. "I'm way ready to have this baby." After a pause she added, "The baby'll be okay, right?"

"When your water breaks prematurely because of an infection, and when that infection's had a few days to take hold—" I searched for the right words, and then decided to give it to her straight. "This is serious, Flora. You're just twenty-two weeks pregnant. If the baby is born now, there's a chance it might not survive."

Tears welled up in Flora's eyes and streaked down her cheeks in thin single lines. She wiped her face, smudging her thick eyeliner into two black blotches under her eyes.

She looked at me. "I just did a little coke, not much. I mean, we had this party going on last weekend and everything. And then my water started coming out but the baby was moving a lot, so I thought everything was okay. I just came in today because the baby hasn't moved much since last night." She shrugged and smiled as if to say, *you know how it is.*

I placed my hand on her arm, the way I've placed my hand a hundred times on other patients' arms.

"I know how scary this must be," I said. I felt disingenuous, cold. I felt that my body was safe, and hers was in danger; that my body was whole, and hers was broken. I sent Flora upstairs to deliver the baby who, it turned out, would not survive.

Finally, when it was almost dusk, I left the clinic.

On my way to the parking garage, I saw, from the corner of my eye, a man lounging against the brick building. As I passed, he scuffed out his smoke and fell into step behind me. We were alone on that side of the hospital. I heard the soft, padded sound of his footfall, his steps echoing mine. Nervous, I walked faster and then started to jog. When he picked up his pace, trailing me, I began to run.

Every time I open the door and see a patient waiting inside—sometimes sitting in a chair, sometimes lying in a bed, sometimes perched on the exam table—I wonder who he or she is, how we are different and, most of all, how we are alike. Working in women's health, I have a professional advantage: I too live in a woman's body and so am subject to that body's strange and wonderful whims. Like many of my patients, I've given birth; I've offered my breasts, laden with milk; I've bled too much and too long; I've had lumps in my breast and surgery to remove them; I've felt the sudden sharp pelvic pains, like a knife in the vagina, that men will never experience. Because I am physically *like* my patients, I can empathize with them and better understand their stories and their symptoms. They believe that I'm less likely to judge them. When I walk into a room, patients sometimes say, "Oh good, I was hoping I'd get a woman."

Still, there is always an invisible, ever-shifting, boundary between a patient and her caregiver, a boundary constructed and maintained by both, for the safety and well-being of both. Our patients, whether in the clinic or on the hospital floors, want us to be like them, yet they also want us to be strong when they are weak, healing when they are hurting, kind when they are overwhelmed, and knowledgeable when they are questioning. As caregivers, we want the same things—and more. Secretly, down deep inside, we want that line between the state of being a "patient" and the state of being "well" to be firmly drawn. Patients exist in bodies that are, for whatever reason, no longer cooperating. We caregivers exist in bodies that are functioning smoothly, allowing us to hum along in our daily tasks. Knowing well the wages of illness, we want to be the ones forever on the outside looking in, peering into patients' ears and eyes and throats, listening to their hearts, palpating their abdomens. We want to be the ones in control, the ones who treat and comfort and then step back, returning safely home to our normal lives.

But what happens when that boundary, that elusive line, disappears, and we are the ones changed by illness, the essence of what is *us* suddenly transformed from the body of a healthy caregiver to the body of a suffering patient? How does being a patient who is also a caregiver, with pockets full of insider information about disease and healing, alter the way we experience our own illnesses, our own physical and mental lapses? What if the converse happens and that line between patient and caregiver becomes a barrier too dense, too thick, too wide to cross, and so instead of acknowledging our similarities, we harden our hearts to our patients' suffering and so also deny our own?

Can we ever truly witness another's suffering? Does reading or writing *about* illness sensitize our responses to our patients—not just touch us in the moment of reading or writing but grab us and shake us and change our lives? As a nurse, I have watched, monitored, recorded, discussed, and charted hundreds of bedside scenarios. As a poet, I've written about some of those same encounters believing that, in the retelling, my interactions with patients and my observations about them might become accessible to readers whose hearts and minds might then open more fully to the experiences of those who suffer. But when I or any other writer put our words *about patients* on the page, no matter how talented we are, how accomplished in imagery and metaphor, we can only represent the original event—the patient's reality—from a distance. Students and providers might be encouraged through literature to see their patients in a new light of understanding, but in the end we are *not* our patients. I don't know how other caregiver-writers feel, but I know that for myself, the only events and emotions I can honestly and accurately witness are my own: what it's like when *I'm* the patient; what it's like to be a nurse bending over the dying; how *my* body feels when it's invaded by instruments, illness, or the examining hands of my own physician. From knowing myself, I hope to come to know my patients.

When I write about my own body and illness, I approach the quest for empathic sensitization—that light of understanding—moving not from theory to experience but from experience to understanding. By revealing my own illnesses and feelings in poems and stories and then sharing my writing, I move from self to other, from the personal to the universal. Then, when confronted with a patient's suffering or with my own feelings of inadequacy in the face of disease, something wonderful happens: the barrier between me and my patient becomes transparent.

When we caregivers let our own diseases or inabilities become the central narrative, we toss a metaphorical stone into the water. The ripples of our personal revelations spread, circle by circle, both into the world and into our own souls, informing and changing the way we experience the greater, universal enterprises of caregiving and care receiving.

Revealing our own bodies and personal failings, however, isn't so easy. We caregivers feel much safer, much less exposed, when we keep our hands in our lab coat pockets and our minds on X-ray results and what time the next patient is scheduled to walk through the door. It's less threatening to write about our patients' bodies than to write about our own—after all, their bodies are undressed and exposed routinely; ours are uniformly veiled and beyond scrutiny.

Writing about ourselves is a two-edged sword. If we reveal our diseased bodies and imperfect minds, we fear others might lose faith in us. If we're patients ourselves, how can we be strong enough to cure others or to work alongside clinical colleagues? Yet if we don't dare name our own illnesses and examine them, we miss the one sure connection we have to witnessing our patients' suffering.

We are most like our patients when our bodies betray us. When they do, we must claim those bodies and celebrate them as *ours*. Even if we think we are somehow different from our patients, when we experience our own illnesses and our own fears, we learn that we are not. Going one step further and writing about our own experiences, we can initiate an important conversation. We might become open to new beliefs. We might change. Which brings me back to that Friday in August, the day I thought my patient, Flora, was in danger, and I was safe.

That morning I had parked my car on the far side of the parking garage. Suddenly terribly afraid of the man who was following me, I began to run. He ran too, his shoes hitting the pavement in time with mine, a twinned *bam bam* that rang sharp and tinny under the garage's huge dome. Although only a few moments had passed, time slowed and I saw Flora's face, how in the clinic she had turned toward me seeking solace, forgiveness, something I did not give her. Considering her as she sat in the exam room, I couldn't imagine myself in her situation. I couldn't imagine my body dirty, invaded, and infected. I'd planted myself safely on the caregiver side of that invisible boundary that separated us, and I'd bricked up the wall so my patient couldn't reach me, and I couldn't reach her.

But running from that man, a man so close I could smell his sweat, I learned how suddenly we can cross that invisible boundary; how we, who give care to others, can in a split second need help and caring ourselves. Heart pounding, mouth dry, body vulnerable and trembling, on that August day, I almost became Flora.

Raped

Alicia sits on the exam table before me, freckles scattered here and there across her nose. Her mouth is bowed. She is twelve, with dark brown hair, pale brown eyes, and a resigned, empty stare.

I sit at her feet on my round rolling stool. I feel as if I am both her nurse and her confessor. Alicia's mother is here too, a small, sad woman who sits in the corner in a straight-back chair. Alicia shivers. She fixes her gaze not on me but on the beige clinic wall.

She tells me that the man came into her apartment when her mother was at work, her sister was shopping. I don't ask, and Alicia doesn't say. Did he speak or cajole? Did he cover her mouth?

When her sister returned, she found Alicia huddled in bed, the sheets rosy with blood.

In the Emergency Room, the doctors opened the rape kit, and Alicia clutched her ears to keep from hearing and covered her mouth to keep from screaming. Under the glare of the overhead light, the physicians inspected her clothes, scraped under her nails, swabbed her throat, her vagina, her rectum, dragged a tiny-toothed comb through her pubic hair. The light revealed a laceration deep in her vagina, so the doctors sutured it—three stitches to join the crimson walls, to hold Alicia together. They drew her blood to test for pregnancy, syphilis, hepatitis, HIV. When the doctors and nurses were finished, Alicia went home, a hollowed-out girl.

Now, two days later, I'm the stranger examining Alicia's healing vagina, her innocent labia. I'm the nurse practitioner ticking off the results: negative pregnancy, negative syphilis, negative hepatitis, negative HIV. I'm the woman who has never been raped, telling Alicia that the still-sharp sutures will dissolve on their own. When, because I don't know what to say, I take hold of her hand, she tells me that the man was a friend of a friend. *I'd met him once before,* she says. *I smiled at him when he walked in.*

Because I'm unable to help Alicia shoulder her grief, resolve her guilt, I call the women's center to make sure the special counselor is on her way. Perhaps she will help Alicia carry the burden of nightmares, the way her thoughts and dreams punish her now, tossing her to and fro.

"I would rather he killed me than raped me," is what Alicia says.

I've lost my words, lost my thoughts, lost everything but touch. I move closer, still holding Alicia's hands in mine, enfolding and warming them.

"Am I still a virgin?" she asks me.

I struggle not to look away. Like Lady Justice, I weigh my patient's words, trying to balance the question and the words *behind* the question. In one hand, a pound of flesh. In the other, the shimmering spirit.

Alicia's mother leans forward. She wears cloth shoes with worn-down heels. She clutches a pocket book in her lap, and under the lackluster clinic lights the patent leather shines like the sun.

"*You* choose to give your virginity, when you marry, when you are in love," I tell her. "In your heart and in your soul, you are still a virgin."

Gracias a Dios, Alicia sighs.

Her mother, nodding, understands the lie.

Alicia tightens her hands in mine. Maybe she believes she will never fall in love.

I help her down from the exam table. I give back her polyester skirt, hand over her white cotton *camisa,* hug her, smooth back her hair.

Alicia's mother and I step out into the hall and wait together beside the closed exam room door. The noises of the clinic assault us. Babies cry, phones ring, beepers squawk, residents rush by.

Not speaking, just holding each other with our eyes, Alicia's mother and I stand guard, fierce and protective, while Alicia dresses.

The Heart's Truth

A young woman, who I will call Susan, had been coming to our hospital clinic for years complaining of a deep pelvic ache that interfered with her intimate relations with her husband. She'd had cultures for infection, Paps, ultrasounds— even an exploratory laparoscopy that discovered no adhesions, no cysts, nothing to explain this troublesome pain.

This particular day, she sat slouched on the exam table. Her short hair was blond and shining, but everything else about her was dark. When I sat down before her, she fixed her gaze on me.

"Sorry I was late," she offered.

"Was it difficult for you to get here?" I asked.

"No. I just wasn't sure why I should bother to come."

"The secretary said that you're still having pelvic pain," I prompted.

"Yes, but everything always comes back negative. My husband thinks this is all in my mind."

I hesitated a moment. "Do *you* believe it's all in your mind? What do you think causes your pain?"

My simple question—had no one asked it before?—released a torrent. Susan began to cry, lifting the sheet and pressing it to her eyes. I thought I could surely guess the reason for her sudden outburst. Maybe she'd been raped or abused, and my question somehow allowed her to acknowledge the pain of those memories. Maybe she was being abused now. I had, ready and waiting, my list of possibilities. But Susan's story surprised me. It also changed the way I practice nursing.

Susan told me that she'd gotten pregnant at sixteen. She told her boyfriend and he told his mother who paid for Susan's abortion. She kept this abortion a secret from her parents and friends. Engaged in her early twenties, she became pregnant again. Even though she wanted to keep this pregnancy, her fiancé didn't think the time was right. Susan had an abortion at his urging. After this termination, Susan became "angry and grouchy." She and her fiancé broke up, and for several years, Susan said, every time she'd see a child about the age her child would have been, she'd weep, hiding her tears, once again, from friends and family. She even calculated when she would have delivered the pregnancy and then, every year, spent that day grieving.

Five years ago, she'd married a "wonderful" man. Even though she wanted to tell him about her two abortions, the time never seemed right.

"After a year or so," Susan said, "he started to talk about our getting pregnant. That's when I started getting this pain. I don't think it's in my head. I think it's in my heart. How can I be a mother, after what I did? What if I become pregnant and something goes wrong?"

I had no easy answer for Susan. I've seen women who choose abortion and have no obvious remorse. I have also seen women who, postabortion, are hounded by grief. Women have told me that they were angry at the incomplete or hasty counseling they received. Some have told me that caregivers tended to minimize the procedure. Other women have told me that they thought their abortion was "in the past," yet suddenly they were experiencing remorse anew, as if it happened only yesterday. Susan mentioned two specific fears: she felt that she didn't deserve to be a mother even when she was choosing to have a baby, and she worried that any wanted pregnancy might now be jinxed. Her abortions were secrets that weighed on her like stones.

Afraid until now to tell anyone these secrets, Susan didn't need more tests— she desperately needed healing. But how could I best help Susan, or any patient, whose lives had been dramatically affected by the choices they'd made? Susan told me that what she wanted most was to feel *forgiven.* She wanted to talk to her husband, telling him her story and trusting in his love and support. But that day, she talked to me, crying until she had no more tears to shed.

Several weeks after our visit, Susan called to tell me that she and her husband were in counseling. She'd done an Internet search and found resources there. Slowly, she was beginning to feel that the weight and the pain of her secret were lifting.

How did Susan change the way I practice nursing? I am, more than ever, sensitive to women who continue to seek help for symptoms even when all tests are negative. Although I always inquire, I don't assume that abuse or rape is the answer. I ask women if they have *anything* in their past that might contribute to depression, grief, or guilt. Then I listen closely with an open mind, not just to the words that play over the surface of a patient's story but to the heart's message behind those words as well.

Watching ER

We nurses share in our patients' joys—the successful operation, the negative scan, the day of discharge—but our days also include crash C-sections, unexpected infections, sudden trauma, and other personal and familial grief. Unlike the smoothly coordinated workings of the TV show *ER* ("We have to crack the chest! Quick, the knife! Rib spreader! There, we're in!"), our jobs consist of a merely human plodding after healing. Some of the time, things don't go so smoothly. Equipment is missing or not working, patients don't spring back to life, and sometimes, at least speaking for myself, I'm just not smart enough. I have to run into the back room and beg for help. Sometimes I have to go into a quiet corner and pray for strength.

"So why," my friends ask me, "*do* you watch *ER*?"

A few years ago, I received a frantic call. My daughter was in the emergency room of a small-town hospital with her ten-month-old daughter. "Can you get here right away?" my daughter pleaded. "She has croup, and I don't think this doctor knows what he's doing!"

It was late at night in the midst of a terrible early spring storm; my husband and I sped the thirty-mile drive, rain and wind making visibility almost impossible. When we rushed into the ER, my granddaughter was lying on a gurney, her body a pale motionless light in the middle of the long black stretcher. A nurse wafted a nebulizer over her face and kept repeating, "Breathe, honey. Breathe." A tall doctor in a blue coat agitated back and forth. When he saw us he grimaced. "Great," he said, "now everyone's here." My daughter pulled me aside. "He's a moonlighter," she said. "It's his first night, and he doesn't know how to intubate a baby. He paged the anesthesiologist on call, but he isn't here and he hasn't answered. The ambulance is on its way from Children's Hospital." Her voice broke. "They said the Life Star helicopter can't fly in this weather. So they're more than an hour away."

On the gurney, my granddaughter stared up at the ceiling, the white steam from the nebulizer condensing on her skin in milky drops. Her eyes were dull and cloudy. The rasp of her breathing mingled with the hiss of the oxygen. All of us—me, the inexperienced physician, the nurse, my husband, my daughter, and my son-in-law—stood by helplessly and listened as our precious baby struggled for air. "Come on, honey," the nurse said. "Stay with us."

I prayed. I prayed hard that the team would arrive from Children's Hospital in time. *And when they do arrive,* I prayed, *let them be skilled.* Let them sweep in and know what to do, their actions a smooth, saving dance. Let them have the right medications and let them know how to thread the tiny breathing tube into my granddaughter's trachea. Let the nurse be kind and alert and one step ahead. Let her take us aside and tell us that everything will turn out fine. Let them keep my granddaughter alive.

An hour later, the team arrived: two pediatric intensive care nurses, two pediatric intensive care residents, and the driver. My granddaughter's airway had narrowed to less than a quarter-inch. The team shooed us out of the room. They told the moonlighting doctor to get out as well. They pulled out their gloves and silver instruments and went to work. A nurse hugged my daughter and explained what was happening. The driver went outside and kept the ambulance motor running. One of the residents, a woman with brown hair and tired brown eyes, tried once, then again, and on the third try inserted the breathing tube into my granddaughter's throat. In the next instant, they were gone. The resident ran beside the stretcher, hand-pumping the Ambu bag. The nurse held the IV bags in the air and pulled the portable crash cart along, keeping her eye on the jagged, racing line that was my granddaughter's heart. The lights of the ambulance twirled as they pulled off into the downpour, my daughter and her husband driving blindly after them. *Lucky,* they told my daughter, and she told me. *If we'd arrived a few minutes later, she wouldn't have made it.*

I still don't know the resident's name or the nurse's. I remember their dark eyes and their swift, sure actions. I envision them sitting beside the small, dusky shape of my granddaughter, pumping the Ambu bag all the way to Children's Hospital in spite of aching hands, in spite of slick and dangerous roads. I know they held my granddaughter to this life until the intensive care staff took over, attaching the respirator that supported her breathing for the three days it took for her croup to subside.

Today my granddaughter is healthy, unaware of her brush with death. By the time she is grown up, *ER* will be long gone, the fantastic and almost unreal episodes—the five-minute open-heart surgery, the rare disease recognized in a flash, the ER doctors and nurses whose ministrations are perfectly timed and perfectly right—banished to reruns on some obscure channel in the middle of the night. Sometimes I imagine that the resident who saved my granddaughter's life graduated and now works in some pediatric intensive care unit. I imagine that the nurse who hugged us all, then ran into the rain alongside the stretcher, is working nearby. Someday I might bump into her in the grocery store. Perhaps she too watches *ER*. Maybe her friends also ask her, "Why?"

My guess is that we watch because, like anyone, we want to trust that doctors and nurses are as well trained and as dedicated as their television counterparts. We want to believe that in an increasingly complex world we have a chance of being saved. We also watch because, as insiders, we know that real doctors and nurses aren't perfect. In our everyday work dramas, we can only imitate those television experts, hoping that once in a while we succeed. Often, we do. When I or my loved ones are patients, I can only pray that someone as talented as that real-life pediatric resident or that real-life intensive care nurse might once again come to rescue us from the storm, their hair flying, their black bag of miracles open and ready.

Feeding the Deer

Only three months after my granddaughter's life-threatening illness, my father died. An only child, I instantly became an orphan. Five months later, I found myself in surgery, undergoing an unexpected, major emergency operation. After I recovered, my mammogram, like a bad joke, came back abnormal, and once again I returned to patient status for a biopsy. Even the benign outcome didn't lift my increasingly dark mood. *So who wouldn't be a little down?* I asked myself and went about my life and my work. But my mind and body twisted in ever-tightening knots.

In the clinic, always feeling just a beat or two removed, I laughed with the residents and nurses. Worse, I felt increasingly distanced from real contact with my patients. Before every exam, I pulled on the latex gloves that protected my patients and me from infection but also blunted the comforting sensation of touch. And there were other restraints: lots of patients and little time; conversations siphoned through translators, deadening the understanding that accompanies real communication; so many hungry or homeless women and not enough resources. If I'd had to name my emotions, I would have said not lonely, but alone. Ineffective.

Driving home, I'd cry, inexplicably moved by radio commercials. In that world, families laughed together at dinner and the laundry always came out spotless. Such innocent happiness was wrenching and unattainable, but it was what I desired for my family, my patients, and myself. At night, I worked hard to finish a book I was writing about women's health and the lessons I'd learned from those same patients. They were brave and resilient. So why couldn't I just snap out of it? What was missing from my life?

I tried to answer that question the way I unravel a patient's symptoms, by ticking off the probable causes. Was it an absence of spirituality? Was I lacking in generosity or expertise as a caregiver? I tried the cures I urged on others: eat well, drink more water, exercise, sleep eight hours, stop listing those undone tasks, and open yourself to the mercy of time.

Then, the winter arrived, and with it, the first big snowstorm. The clinic closed, and I stayed home, thankful to have one day in which no patient called my name, no woman sat crying before me. Drinking tea and isolated in my numbing sadness, I watched three deer claw at the snow looking for food. Their stomachs were drawn up with hunger. When they sensed me standing at the window, they lifted their snow-clotted muzzles and sprinted away, thin-muscled and ephemeral.

The next morning, I drove to Agway and came home with five fifty-pound bags of deer food, a sticky, grainy concoction that resembled the sweet feed I once scooped out for my children's pony. I filled a bucket and carried it to the edge of the driveway. The sweet feed made molasses-smelling pockets in the white drifts.

Soon, eleven deer were arriving every morning at 6 a.m., some with fawns trembling in their speckled coats. I got up before my husband, pulled on boots, and threw a coat over my bathrobe. Going into the dawn, I felt as naked and vulnerable as the women I examined in the clinic. Cold air stung my bare legs and fluttered up under my nightgown. The deer snorted and jumped back, hungry, waiting for me to dump the sweet feed and leave.

Day by day, the sun's angle changed. The skies were pink or gray and, most mornings, clouds blew like rags across the sunrise. By nightfall, the deer gathered again in quiet circles. My interaction with them seemed elemental, involving neither obligation nor expectation. I could offer my full bucket twice a day, but I had no control over how many would come forward and eat or how, if what I gave wasn't enough, they would help themselves to survive. I was, for the first time in a long time, content.

In April, when green, spear-headed shoots began to emerge, I stopped feeding the deer. All winter, I'd felt exposed and innocent, unable to shield myself from sound or smell, from the small nuances of weather, or from the realization that I could only do so much, a small trespasser with her bucket. But I could do something. It seems, in retrospect, such a simple thing.

Every year, I feed the deer, imagining that they need me. Every spring, women arrive at the clinic, crowds of them newly pregnant and waiting in the hallways for information and reassurance, for someone like me to share their happiness.

When Their Rhythms Become Mine

Working as a nurse practitioner, serving uninsured women and teenagers, I've gotten really good at doing first exams. I even have something of a reputation: fifteen-year-old girls come in for an appointment and say, "You did my friend's first exam and she said it wasn't too awful." Some of the nurses steer the first exams my way as well. When she hands me a chart, a nurse might say, "I'm glad it's you. It's the patient's first pelvic and she looks scared to death."

When I was younger and horseback riding was my passion, I was also good at calming skittish horses. I couldn't get the sluggish mare moving, no matter how I kicked and prodded, but when I encountered the wild-eyed ones something mysterious happened. If a frightened chestnut jigged sideways or took off running, I would let my weight sink into the saddle, settling back as if nothing could dislodge me, and the horse's rhythm became mine. The animal's muscular energy flowed into my body and rose up through my spine until I could feel myself softening and accepting. As I slowed my breathing and let myself linger one beat behind the horse's movement, a peaceful calm settled over us. Little by little, my body and the horse's body became one.

The young women I see in the clinic are wild-eyed too, like foals weaned too early from their mothers. These girls prance in for their initial appointments, all nerve and pretense. Sometimes they want a Pap test. Other times they think something is wrong and want to be checked. Then, behind the closed exam room door, when they shed their clothes and pull on their johnny coats, they become frightened, unpredictable, and lonely. I've learned how to place my hand on a girl's arm, just for a moment, allowing some of her fear to escape, just as that good nurse once placed her hand on my arm, saving me. I've learned how to drape a young woman's body so that she isn't exposed, and I know how to do an exam in a controlled, calm manner, letting the patient's rhythm become, for that brief span of time, my rhythm too. Because my body is like my patients' bodies, we can chance the mysteries of this exam.

At the end of my riding lessons, I'd return to my suburban home where I'd have a good lunch of hot soup and sandwiches. My parents loved me. But many of my patients, abandoned by their mothers, come to the clinic for their first appointments alone. Some of them have been raped by their friends, brothers, or uncles. Jittering from one relationship to another, many of the girls I see have chlamydia, herpes, abnormal Pap tests, and other diseases. They smoke, sometimes they use drugs, and long before they are old enough to drive or buy cigarettes, they become sexually active and blind to the consequences: sad lives, infertility, abortion, grief, cervical cancer, fractured bodies.

I was never afraid when I rode horses, not worried about falling off or breaking bones. But when I first came to work in the clinic, I was afraid of these girls, tough girls with tattoos and loud mouths who shouted at each other in the waiting room and sometimes walked out on me. "Bitch," one of them called me once, spitting the words at my feet.

After a few years in women's health, just when I wondered if I should give up and work somewhere else, I met seventeen-year-old Lourdes, a tall, hazel-eyed beauty who came for her first exam. She barely spoke English, and her Spanish was too rapid-fire for me to follow. "*Mas despacio,*" I said, and she glared and hammered on, thrusting the edge of her hand at me when I didn't understand. At that first visit, I discovered she had three sexually transmitted diseases— chlamydia, herpes, and a nasty case of trichomoniasis. Although Lourdes was furious when I told her about the infections, and even though we were hardly able to communicate, she kept coming back. At some visits I'd see that her thin arms were bruised—ragged patches in purple, red, and blue—but when I asked who was hurting her, she'd growl and show the whites of her eyes. Once, when her vagina was raw, disks of skin slicked away like the shiny wounds left by rug or rope burns, she lifted her heel from the exam table stirrup and kicked my arm as I tried to examine her. When I called the social worker, Lourdes swore, threatened me, and ran out of the clinic.

The last time I saw Lourdes, her back was scarred, the flesh blistered into small round puckers. I asked if her family practiced the folk art of "cupping," attaching hot suction cups to Lourdes's skin in order to call out the poisons.

"*No, no,*" she said. "*Mi papa fumas.*"

My father smokes.

Maybe it was the horror of the picture in my mind—Lourdes's father grinding out his cigarettes on her cinnamon-colored skin—or maybe it was the way she spoke matter-of-factly, as if she were simply recounting some common symptom. It might have been my frustration at being unable to reach or to help her, but whatever the cause, tears came to my eyes. I sat looking up at Lourdes. She looked down, and I waited for her to laugh. *La blancita,* she'd nicknamed me. Little white girl.

Minutes went by. I didn't know what to do and, gut sick as if I'd been punched in the stomach, I couldn't speak. I took a breath and wiped my cheeks dry. For once, Lourdes too was speechless, perhaps overcome with the enormity of her own suffering and only able to realize it when she saw it reflected in my eyes.

Like any abused creature, she had constructed a defense of wary anxiety, quick reflexes, and a guise of self-sufficiency. And I, somewhere along the way, had forgotten in my adulthood what I'd known so well in my youth—how to meld and merge into another creature's wildness, and in so doing, share the burden of apprehension.

Lourdes began to cry and, once loosed, her cries rang out. When I held her arms to steady her, she sensed that I couldn't be dislodged. Little by little, her body memories and mine became one, and when calm at last settled over us, we did the necessary work. The police came. The notes I'd written in Lourdes's chart and the scars on her body became evidence. A representative from the women's shelter escorted Lourdes to a safe haven and there, at last, she was free.

Since then, I've often wondered what happened on that particular day to enable Lourdes to tell her story, in spite of our language barrier and in spite of all the other times I'd asked how I could assist her. I can only guess that it was the combination of my sorrow and my silence; for once I wasn't a do-good nurse who pried for answers but simply another woman willing to share the heart's grief and go along for the ride.

I Believe in Grief

I believe in grief. Almost every day, when I walk into the hospital, I hear crying, moaning, or wailing: a young woman has miscarried, an elderly widower is holding his wife's belongings, a mother stands guard over her badly burned child.

Once I would have rushed to comfort these people. Uncomfortable myself with their grief, I'd want to ease their sadness with my cheer and consolation. I'd hug a patient and tell her to "try to get pregnant next month." I'd reassure the widower, telling him, "Your wife had a long life." I'd enter the burned child's room in Intensive Care with a smile rather than encouraging the mother to weep in my arms.

When my own mother died I was terrified, confused about how I was expected to act. Was I allowed to be the grieving daughter, or should I be the competent, grief-denying professional? I held my mother's wrist, counting her pulse as it slowed. After her last breath, I rang for the nurse. Heart pounding, I waved good-bye to my mother, her gray hair bright against the sheets, and said, "Bye Mom!" in the cheery voice I'd practiced all my life. I didn't know then that I could have climbed into bed and held her, or that I should have wailed when she was gone.

It wasn't until I had stayed with many dying patients and, finally, with my dying father, that I allowed myself to grieve—for my parents, for those lost patients, for all their loved ones who, as I once did, held back their tears. At my father's death I cried like a child, not caring that I made the gulping noises of unrestrained mourning. Now, years later, I know that it is both necessary and human for us to wallow, each in our own way, in grief.

I no longer comfort others with false cheer. In the hospital, where my encounters with patients are ever more distanced by sterile gloves, computer protocols, and the pressures of time, one way I can still be present is during their moments of grief. I don't encourage anyone to move on, to replace, to remarry, or put the photos or the memories away. Grief must be given its time.

I believe that both the caregivers and the cared-for should be free to scream and cry and fall to the floor—if not actually, then at least in the heart. I believe that grief, fully expressed, will change over time into something less overpowering, even granting us a new understanding, a kind of double vision that comprehends both the beauty and fragility of life.

When I grieve, when I stand by others as they grieve, even in the midst of seemingly unbearable sorrow, grief becomes a way to honor life; a way to cling to every fleeting, precious moment of joy.

Human Feelings, Human Experiences

I think a lot about the meaning of words. Years ago, listening to the news, we heard the phrase "shock and awe" used to describe the massive, initial bombing of Iraq, a display of might and power meant to shock Saddam Hussein into surrender. Then, when his soldiers didn't immediately give up, some announcers talked about how "shocked" they were by Iraqi resolve.

We nurses are no strangers to shock or to awe. Surely we have a special understanding of how disaster and illness can shock us, whether we are patient or provider. Certainly we've also experienced firsthand the phenomenon we call awe, what my dictionary describes as "the mixed emotion of reverence, dread, and wonder." Maybe we've been awed by a patient's bravery. Maybe we've been patients ourselves, shocked by illness and amazed at both the fragility and the resilience of the human body. I'd like to think it's our capacity to experience shock and awe that enables us to interact humanely with patients, to touch their lives and enrich our own.

But shock and awe take their toll. How often have we thought that we couldn't stand to witness any more suffering? How many times have we been overwhelmed by the roadblocks we must negotiate in order to help a patient? And what about the joy and poignancy that is also a part of our profession? What do we do with the mixed emotions that come our way—pain, helplessness, happiness, the sense of loss as well as the recognition of transcendence?

I have a friend, a nurse, who recently took up photography. Her black-and-white photos are evocative: gravestones in snow; the shadows of teenagers loitering on the streets; the side-glance of an elderly woman. She says that looking through an artistic lens instead of a clinical one renews her spirit and brings her comfort. Another nurse friend is an actress. When she plays a role, she becomes, for a time, another person. This helps her understand the narratives of her patients' lives from alternative points of view. When another nurse friend was diagnosed with breast cancer, her response was to paint her emotions, documenting them on canvas. My choice is creative writing; poetry and stories that give voice to my fears about death, suffering, abandonment, and loneliness, as well as to my celebrations of birth, relationship, and love. There's something about the act of putting words on the page that helps me look again at my experiences. Often, I write about moments of shock and awe. Always, I wonder what other nurses, other providers, are doing to help themselves cope.

The author Saul Bellow said that poetry helps "human feelings, human experiences, the human form and face, recover their proper place—the foreground." Of course, no nurse or doctor would ever argue against having "the human form and face" in the foreground. That's why we went into health care. At the same time, many caregivers believe they're not creative—after all, so much of our time and energy go into achieving clinical excellence.

Doctors have realized the importance of using literature as a way to balance the imagination and the scientific for quite some time. Many medical schools incorporate the humanities into their curriculum. Many physicians publish their poems and stories, allowing readers to discover another side of medicine, one that wrestles creatively with the shock and awe patients and their caregivers know so well.

Many nurses are writing too, beautifully, about their work—and yet, as a profession, nursing has not yet embraced literature as an essential part of nursing education.

Let me extend both a challenge and an invitation. The challenge is to nursing educators: please, please incorporate the arts and humanities into nursing programs. Let's not miss this opportunity. Give our students a way to dialogue creatively, helping them use the arts to make sense of all they will encounter in the changing world of health care. And if you already teach humanities in your program, get the word out. Let others know how to use the arts to enhance nursing education.

If you're a student nurse, ask your instructors to talk about how nursing is represented in literature, not the clinical writings but the poems, novels, and stories. If you're a practicing nurse, seek out what other nurses have to say. We are a privileged group, and we have much to contribute. We see and do what few others are permitted. When we write about our work or read what others have written, we open our hearts. We make emotional sense of our profession, and we honor our patients and ourselves.

Finally, here's the invitation—to nurses, to patients, to all caregivers. When you have time, try this writing exercise. You can do this by yourself or in a group. It will unsettle and inform you, and it may also become a vessel into which you can pour images and emotions, looking again at your experiences as a care provider or a patient.

Ready?

WRITING ABOUT A ROOM IN WHICH SOMETHING HAPPENED

1) First, get comfortable. Take a deep breath. Spend a few minutes remembering something that happened when you were caring for others or being cared for, something that moved you or frightened you or changed you in some way. Often some event will pop immediately into your mind—that's the one you want.

2) Put yourself *back* into this event and into the room where this happened. Who was there? Where were people standing or sitting or lying in the room? What did you smell, hear, touch? What kind of light was in the room? What did you feel on your skin? Concentrate on your senses. Reimagine every moment of this event. Let your mind be like a camera, panning the room, noticing every detail. Move through the room slowly.

3) When you see the scene in your mind's eye and recall the *emotions* of this event vividly (even if you don't remember all the details), write down seven words that capture what you were feeling then (or what you are feeling now).

4) Without pausing, without giving yourself a chance to censure your writing or change your mind, write about what happened, using those seven words in the writing. Write quickly, as if you were there again. Don't worry about spelling or grammar. Don't worry about your writing being "good."

5) If you get stuck, go back again to the room, to the event. Enter it again and then keep writing. You will know when it's time to stop, and you will most certainly be surprised by what you have written. You'll discover how creative you are, how creative we all are.

6) You can share your writing with others if this has been a group exercise. If not, you can keep your writing hidden in a drawer and peek at it now and then. If it's solid, if it seems to have something to say to others, consider revising it when you are feeling more emotionally distanced from the event. In the cool light of revision, you can fix your grammar and find strong verbs to replace weak verbs. You can change patient and staff names and descriptions to protect their privacy. You can take this baby, newly born, and clean it up. Then you can present it to the world.

7) Maybe you can even publish it. There are many nursing and medical journals looking for poems and stories by patients, nurses, and other caregivers.

Literary journals, ones not associated with health care, are also very interested in what we have to say. We inhabit a world unknown to others. But publishing is not necessarily the goal. If this exercise has let you relive a health care moment deeply, if it has brought you release or joy or a memory to cherish, if it has captured for you human feelings and human experiences, then its work is done.

Conscious Suffering

"To be competent to speak of pain is to speak of pain that isn't yours. This requires experiencing pain that is yours."

—SHARON CAMERON IN *BEAUTIFUL WORK: A MEDITATION ON PAIN*

I'm sick. I'm so sick I haven't gone to work for days. Staying home is something I rarely do. Usually I manage to drag myself in, despite a runny nose, headache, back pain.

Not this time.

I'm so sick I'm *in bed* in my pajamas and fuzzy robe. So sick I haven't made it downstairs to turn on my computer and must instead write in my scribbly hand on a yellow legal pad and hope that, later, when I'm able, I can decipher these scratchings and type them into words.

Because I'm a nurse, illness is part of my life, my daily bread, my soul-work. For more years than I care to remember I have cared for others. But now, I'm the one suffering.

Usually, I try not to get carried away at the onset of a personal illness. Instead, treating myself as if I were my own patient, I take a history and then a body inventory. When did this illness first begin? What, exactly, are the symptoms? I'm on the alert for the serious symptoms, the ones that almost shout *emergency room,* things like shortness of breath, chest pain, fever of 103 degrees, unrelenting abdominal pain, and the like. For the past three days, I've been anxiously taking and retaking my history and body inventory.

Headache? At first, it was mild but persisted in spite of Advil. Sinuses? Not a touch of congestion. Throat? For the first several days I felt as if ground glass had been mashed into the tissues of my upper pharynx. When I looked with a flashlight, saying *ahhhh* like I ask patients to say, I could see that my throat was beefy red. My throat, as patients say, was killing me.

Deep slow breath with mouth open. Lungs fully expanding? Well, almost. The virus had insinuated itself from throat to lungs, creeping down my main stem bronchus and spreading itself over the surface mucosa of my bronchial tree just as fine beach sand sticks to moist skin. The tissues scritched and scraped with my every breath. Whenever I took a breath, I felt as if I were a hundred feet underwater.

Within days, my symptoms crescendoed, yet for a while I functioned, as we women do, watering plants, grocery shopping, making lunches, and going to work in the clinic as I have for years. Then, at work on day four of the still-on-my-feet part of this illness, I was suddenly struck with that peculiar and horrible feeling, as if someone had pulled a plug in my ankles and all my energy was draining out, streaming from my ankle bones in twin rivulets and soaking into the already stained clinic carpeting. One minute I was smiling and talking to a patient. The next moment I felt myself deflating, becoming pale. My heart raced. There was a high-pitched buzzing in my ears. What was wrong with me? As soon as I'd thought that thought, I began coughing, a spasm so intense, so prolonged I couldn't catch my breath or talk. While horrified hospital employees stood by, helpless, I waved my hand to signal *I'm okay*. When I finally mouthed the word *water*, three people scurried as one to fetch me a Styrofoam cup of warm tap water. Tiny sips seemed to calm things down.

Then I felt faint. I flushed steamy hot and bright red, partly from embarrassment and partly from fear. I felt really, really sick. "I have to go home," I said. It was barely an hour and a half into my shift, but everyone nodded, happy to have whatever germ I was harboring go home with me.

Once in the parking garage, key in the ignition, I wasn't sure I could drive. My vision seemed to brighten and dim, alternately, and my legs were shaking. I kept coughing, on the brink of another spasm, which frightened me. What if I coughed so hard I ran off the road or caused an accident? What if I managed to pull over but couldn't stop coughing? What if I passed out in my car? Stuck between *here in the parking garage* and *there at home, there* seemed a better place to be; I decided to chance it. When I at last pulled into my garage, all in one piece and with no dents in the car, I felt wildly grateful. I walked straight into the bedroom, stepped out of my clothes and into my pajamas and robe, and, folding back the covers, got in, and collapsed against my two propped pillows.

I was sure that there was something terribly wrong. If only I could figure out what it was, then I could understand it, know it, cure it—control it. My body was light, as if it was trying to levitate from the bed. I was dizzy, and the room seemed extra bright. My steady pulse didn't speak of anxiety or an impending swoon. Instead, I felt *something* shift in the core of my being. It was this *something*—a feeling no doubt familiar to patients and yet not documented in any of the anatomy and physiology books—that made me think, as I sat there in bed staring at the blank reflective face of the TV across the room, that I might actually be dying.

When we're young and sick we rarely think we might be dying. In our thirties and forties, a brief virus or bacterial illness might perplex and worry us, but still we hardly ever think that this could be it, the fatal blow. When we humans cross the line into our fifties and sixties, however, illness takes on a different shape, a different beat. Even a simple virus might be, our shadow half reminds us, the beginning of the end. Maybe, we think, we don't have a simple virus but avian flu. Maybe the cough isn't just bronchitis or even a mild pneumonia but that unusual and fatal pulmonary condition discussed on TV last night. Maybe the stomach bug is really the blocked and nonfunctioning bowel, soon to gangrene. Maybe the pain in the breast is the warning of the lump that will be the cancer that will bring, sooner or later, the inevitable end.

I have, I think, a solid intellectual understanding of mortality. I see the seasons slide by, and I've sat with enough dying patients to understand that death comes to us all—leafy tree or human being. I believe too that I'm deeply aware of the state of being we call suffering and how suffering can exist separate from or conjoined with illness and death. I have suffered myself, physically, and I have, as we all have, suffered emotionally. I have held sobbing parents whose children are ill, and I've comforted patients suffering with other losses—blindness, amputation, paralysis. I've had my own serious illnesses and my own losses and so have contemplated, often, the ways in which we will all eventually lose everything that we are, everything that is ours on this earth. Like everyone, I have cried at the thought of someday leaving behind family and friends and this beautifully complex world.

But during this particular illness I learned something else about suffering. Not with my mind but with my body and, dare I say it in our secular age, most of all with my soul. During those days in bed, laid low, I came to understand that illness is, in its own annoying way, a gift. This recognition occurred when, alone, exhausted and frightened, I stopped listing and evaluating my symptoms and simply sank down into the *reality* of sickness. I gave in to suffering, especially to the horrible *something* that came in waves, sweeping over me—the odd lightness of my body, the illumination and paling of my vision, that high-pitched hum in my ears, as if my soul were trying to drag itself from my flesh, stretched out by some invisible hand, pulled taut like dough is pulled by women in the kitchen, laughing and talking, making bread.

As soon as I let go of being the nurse, of believing that I might be always in control, I recalled something I'd read many, many years ago. The words, clipped out of an article about Cardinal Cooke's illness and death had been forgotten, but now they came back to me entire: "He wants this to be purposeful. He wants his suffering to be a beautiful gift for others. Catholics believe that suffering can be dedicated to a purpose, including the salvation of the souls of others." Reading this paragraph years ago, I'd understood with my mind but not with my flesh. Maybe I hadn't been a nurse long enough. Maybe I hadn't yet seen so many others suffer or suffered enough myself. But now, during this brief illness, I *incorporated* the truth of those words—I took them into my body. Their import struck me like lightning. *Of course,* I said, and then simply opened the door for whatever it was, this suffering. I beckoned it in, I claimed it, and then I gave it away.

I let my body relax, sinking into the pillows. I closed my eyes and offered my suffering, this frightening about-to-die feeling, for the good of another, a close friend, in order that her suffering might be lessened. This small act, this tiny gift, accomplished something astounding. I may never know if my friend has suffered less because of my offering. I do know that my suffering assumed new shape, new import. The sicker I felt, the more I suffered, the more I had to give away, as if each symptom, each moment of discomfort or fear was a gold coin. Instead of being anxious about my inability to feel better, I accepted my situation as a gift and then passed that gift along, currency to reduce another's debt. In bed, unable to read or think or watch television, I thought of all the other times when my suffering had been greater. What a shame I had wasted those moments by hoarding them to myself, by cataloging and trying to reason them away! What a shame that, once, I had mentally chided a patient for "giving in" to illness when I wanted him to fight. Now I understood that one does fight, does cling to life precisely by accepting suffering and actively, consciously, using it.

All this time, standing alongside suffering patients, perhaps helping them endure, perhaps not, I had never acknowledged suffering as useful—other than giving a nod to that old saw that says suffering makes our moments of joy more potent, which is true enough but not the whole truth. This particular illness, in the end a minor one, nevertheless brought me up short. For a few days, I entered a realm I hadn't truly entered before.

Was that rushing wind simply a physical symptom that might be explained away as the sound of blood pumped by the beating heart, the effects of fever or the machinations of anxiety? Good nurse that I am, I know that it was not. The noise in my head and the sudden recognition of suffering as opportunity was the voice of my soul.

So ended my essay, originally, and so, two weeks later, ended my illness. But something happened more recently that seems a part of this and so must be added on.

I have gone to the local post office to get my mail. Walking in, feeling better but still weak, I see a man I know. He looks terrible. There is an off-color cast to his skin, and the blue circles beneath his eyes tell me he has not been sleeping. Still, he greets me with a big smile and a hug. *Are you all right?* I query. *I'm fine,* he says. *I'm healthy myself, but I have two friends for whom I'm suffering. What else,* he asks me, *is the human heart for?*

Indeed. I'm a nurse. I know exactly what he means.

Afterword

When I was not quite a year old, my mother's dormant tuberculosis flared and my father, just home from Italy at the end of World War II, was suffering from terrible nightmares—what we'd now call post-traumatic stress disorder. My parents decided I'd be better off in a healthier environment and so sent me to live with their best friends, a couple with two children of their own, a boy and a girl.

I became their second daughter and the baby of the family. As months went by (they would write me many years later), I seemed to forget my parents. Nevertheless, I was not quite at home in my new family. In a photo from that time I'm sitting on my surrogate mother's lap, straining toward the camera as if I might catch sight of someone I know in the lens. She holds me tight and her two children smile at me, but I'm flailing my arms, frowning, trying to escape.

After I learned to talk, after living with this other family for almost as long as I'd lived with my parents, my mother and father came to reclaim me. Once again, I switched families. My mother's health had improved; my father had a good job and seemed to be coping with his nightmares. My parents told me I readjusted quickly. However, for a long time I couldn't tolerate the slightest separation. If my mother turned the corner in a grocery store, out of sight only for a moment, I would fall to the floor screaming, thinking she was gone forever.

Once I was reunited with my family, my childhood was for the most part happy and constant, yet I never quite got over the sense that someone I loved might, at any minute, disappear. Encouraged by my father and compelled by what might be called my "imagination of disaster"—a trait we shared—I began to write stories and poems, a perfect way to reexperience and make sense of the ephemeral world and my place within it. Then I grew up and I became a nurse. No wonder—we nurses are masters of the fine art of separation.

At the end of this small collection of essays, I find myself practicing this fine art once again, saying good-bye to the hospital and to the women's health clinic, the place I've worked for almost seventeen years. Promoted to management a few years ago and so rarely seeing patients, I simply couldn't stay. While many nurses flourish in administrative roles, I couldn't let go of patient care—I just can't stop being *a nurse*. And so I begin yet another adventure, a position as a nurse practitioner in a new institution, a new setting. My patients will be men and women in the early and sometimes difficult years of adulthood. They will have much to teach me.

Interestingly, I find that when I'm not seeing patients, it's a struggle for me to write. It seems that for me, nursing and writing have become, over the years, inextricably bound. That intimate connection that links us, human to human, is essential both to my vocation and my avocation.

For me, nursing is intimate, tactile, spiritual, and utterly unlike any other way we humans have of communicating with one another. Nursing is not mothering and yet it shares some of mothering's traits. Nursing is not doctoring, even though nurses are as essential to a patient's well-being and recovery as physicians. Nursing is neither friendship nor love, yet many nurses do love their patients, just as patients often love their nurses. And in nursing—just as in mothering, friendship, or love—we must, sooner or later, confront the reality of separation, even when that separation is accompanied by joy.

When we care for patients, our ministrations are akin to praise: we acknowledge even the smallest human detail, in a sense blessing the patient for the journey to come. We marvel at the secrets of the body. We honor the body, for somewhere inside it dwells the soul. How many times, caring for a patient, does a nurse stand in silence, letting her hands convey what speech cannot? How many times does a patient, in the company of his nurse, find that words are unnecessary? We nurses spend time with our patients, thankful for the opportunity to serve in such an uncluttered and honest way, sharing the moment when two human beings stand together honoring the gift of life.

We nurses tend our patients—sometimes they leave us, and sometimes we leave them. No matter the outcome, we are privileged to become the guardians of their memories. We hide these memories in our pockets. We save them in our hearts. Sometimes, we write about them.

Acknowledgments

My appreciation to the editors of the following journals, anthologies, and texts in which versions or sections of these essays first appeared:

Advance for Nurse Practitioners: "Twenty-four Hours in the Life of a Nurse Practitioner" (as "Memories I Carry with Me: Twenty-four Hours in the Life of a Nurse Practitioner")

American Journal of Nursing: "The Heart's Truth" (as "The Pain: Susan's Guilt"), "First, Do No Harm" (as "Milagros")

Lumina: "Washing Mrs. Cardiff s Feet"

Medhuntersmagazine.com: "Breaking Bad News," "Raped" (as "About a Girl"), "Feeding the Deer," "Conscious Suffering" (as "A Nurse Experiences Suffering"), "First Night in Charge"

Nursing Education Perspectives: "The Other Side of Illness," "The Evening Back Rub," "Weekly Rounds"

Rattle: "Nursing and the Word"

RN Magazine: "Beyond Scientific Explanation" (as "Strange Happenings"), "When Their Rhythms Become Mine" (as "Tough Girl, Tough Patient")

Stories of Illness and Healing: Women Write Their Bodies (Kent State University Press): "Becoming Flora" (as "Becoming Flora: When the Illness Narrative is Our Own")

The Teacher's Body: Embodiment, Authority and Identify in the Academy (State University of New York Press): "Body Teaching"

"Hearing the Stories behind our Patients' Words" was first presented as a talk for the Humanities Hour at the University of Maryland at Baltimore

"Being at the Bedside of the Dying" and sections of the Afterword were adopted from commentaries that first appeared in *The Poetry of Nursing: Poems and Commentaries of Leading Nurse-Poets* (Kent State University Press)

"The Other Side of Illness" also appeared in *Intensive Care: More Poetry and Prose by Nurses* (University of Iowa Press)

"I Believe in Grief" first appeared as a commentary on National Public Radio's *I Believe* series